The Home Health Aide Handbook

Jetta Fuzy, RN, MS

Adapted from Dr. William Leahy's
Providing Home Care: A Textbook for Home Health Aides

SECOND EDITION

06-2102

Hartman Publishing Inc.   *hartman*online.com

Acknowledgments

MANAGING EDITOR
Susan Alvare

INTERIOR AND COVER DESIGNER
Kirsten Browne

ILLUSTRATOR/PAGE LAYOUT
Thaddeus Castillo

PROOFREADER
Suzanne Wegner

PHOTOGRAPHY
Art Clifton/Dick Ruddy/Susana Marks

SALES/MARKETING
Gailynn Garberding/Debbie Rinker

CUSTOMER SERVICE
Yvonne Gillam/Kim Williams

A heartfelt thanks goes to our resourceful reviewers, Lyla Berry, RN, MA and Barbara M. Jennings, RN, for their valuable suggestions.

Copyright Information

Notice to Readers

Though the guidelines and procedures contained in this text are based on consultations with healthcare professionals, they should not be considered absolute recommendations. The instructor and readers should follow employer, local, state, and federal guidelines concerning healthcare practices. These guidelines change, and it is the reader's responsibility to be aware of these changes and of the policies and procedures of his or her healthcare agency.

The publisher, author, editors, and reviewers cannot accept any responsibility for errors or omissions or for any consequences from application of the information in this book and make no warranty, expressed or implied, with respect to the contents of the book. The publisher does not warrant or guarantee any of the products described herein or perform any analysis in connection with any of the product information contained herein.

Gender Usage

This textbook utilizes the pronouns "he," "his," "she," and "hers" interchangeably to denote care team members and clients.

Table of Contents

Defining Home Health Services

Foundation of Client Care

III

Understanding Your Clients

IV

Client Care

v

Special Clients, Special Needs

8

VI

Home Management and Nutrition

VII

Caring for Yourself

VIII

Appendix

Welcome

to Hartman Publishing's Home Health Aide Handbook.

We hope you will happily place this little reference book into your purse, backpack, or your home care visit bag and leave it there so you will have it available at all times as you go about your day-to-day duties as a home health aide. This handbook will serve as a quick but comprehensive reference tool for you to use from client to client.

Features and Benefits

This book is a valuable tool for many reasons. For home health aides, it includes all the procedures you learned in your training program, plus references to abbreviations, medical terms, care guidelines for specific diseases, and an appendix for you to write down important names and phone numbers. For certified nursing assistants moving to home care, we've included information on making the transition from facilities to homes. In addition, this book contains all of the federal requirements for home health aides, so it can also be used in a basic training program.

We have divided the book into eight parts and assigned each part its own colored tab, which you'll see at the top of every page.

DEFINING HOME HEALTH SERVICES

FOUNDATION OF CLIENT CARE

UNDERSTANDING YOUR CLIENTS

CLIENT CARE

SPECIAL NEEDS, SPECIAL CLIENTS

HOME MANAGEMENT AND NUTRITION

CARING FOR YOURSELF

APPENDIX

You'll find blue key terms throughout the text. Explanations for these terms are in the Glossary in the Appendix of this book. Common Disorders, Guidelines and Observing and Reporting are also colored for easy reference. Procedures are indicated with a black bar. There is also an index in the back of the book, and on the back cover, you'll see a more detailed explanation of how to use the color tabs. We will be updating this guide periodically, so don't hesitate to let us know what you would like to see in the next handbook we publish.

CONTACT US AT:
Hartman Publishing, Inc., 8529 Indian School Rd NE, Albuquerque, NM 87112. Phone (505) 291-1274, Fax (505) 291-1284
Web: www.**hartman**online.com, E-mail: orders@**hartman**online.com

I
Defining Home Health Services

1. Home Health Care

Home health aides provide assistance to the recovering or chronically ill, the elderly, and to those who provide care and sometimes need relief from the physical and emotional stress of caregiving. Many home health aides also work in assisted living facilities, which provide independent living in a homelike group environment, with professional care available as needed. As advances in medicine and technology extend the lives of people with chronic illnesses, the number of people needing health care will increase. The need for home health aides will also increase.

Payers and Providers

Agencies pay you from payments they receive from the following payers:

- Insurance company
- Health maintenance organization (HMO)
- Preferred provider organization (PPO)
- Medicare
- Medicaid
- The individual client or family

The Centers for Medicare & Medicaid Services (CMS), formerly the Health Care Finance Administration (HCFA), is a department of the government that regulates the Medicare program at the federal level.

Major changes have taken place in the way agencies are paid for care their staff provides. Medicare now pays agencies a fixed fee for a 60-day period of care based on a client's condition. If the cost of providing care exceeds the payment, the agency loses money. If the care provided costs less than the payment, they make money. For these reasons, home health agencies must pay great attention to costs. And because all payers monitor the quality of care provided, the way work is documented or recorded is very important.

CMS's new payment system for home care is called the "Prospective Payment System."

Purpose of Home Care

Perhaps the most important reason for health care in the home is that most people who are ill or disabled feel more comfortable when they are cared for at home with their families and loved ones nearby. Health care in familiar surroundings improves mental and physical well-being. It has proven to be a major factor in the healing process.

2. Agency Structure

Clients who need home care are referred to a home health agency by their doctors. They may also be referred by a hospital discharge planner, a social services agency, the state or local department of public health, the welfare office, a local Agency on Aging, or a senior center. Clients and family members can also choose an agency that meets their needs. Once an agency is chosen and the doctor has made a referral, a staff member performs an assessment of the client. This determines how the client's care needs can best be met. The home environment will also be evaluated to determine whether it is safe for the client.

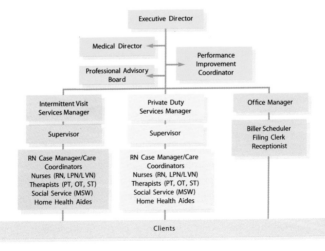

Home health agencies employ many home health aides (HHAs) and certified nursing assistants (CNAs). Services provided may include nursing care, specialized therapy, specific medical equipment, pharmacy and intravenous (IV) products, and personal care. The services provided depend on the size of the agency. Small agencies may provide basic nursing care, personal care, and housekeeping services. Larger agencies may provide speech, physical, and occupational therapies and medical social work. All home health agencies have professional staff who make decisions about what care and services are needed.

3. HHA's Role

A home health aide may be assigned to "make a visit." That means to spend a certain number of hours each day or week with a client to provide personal care and housekeeping services. While the supervisor or case manager develops the assignments and client care plans, input from all members of the care team is needed. In home care, all HHAs are under supervision of the skilled professional assigned to the case: a registered nurse, a physical therapist, or a speech therapist.

In some ways, working as a home health aide is similar to working as a nursing assistant or nurse's aide. In addition to the basic medical procedures and many of the personal care procedures, your job will also include:

- **Housekeeping.** The amount of housekeeping duties you have will depend primarily on how much time you are scheduled to work with an individual client. Tasks must be prioritized according to the assignment description, the client's needs, and what time permits.

- **Family contact.** You will frequently work with the family as a team, encouraging them to participate as much as possible in meeting the goals of the care plan.

- **Independence.** You will work independently as an HHA. Your supervisor will monitor your work, but you will spend most of your hours working with clients without direct supervision.

- **Communication.** Communication skills are important. You must keep yourself informed of changes in the client care plan. You must also keep others informed of changes you observe in the client and the client's environment.

- **Transportation.** You will have to get yourself safely from one client's home to another. You will need to have a dependable car or know how to use public transportation.
- **Safety.** You must be aware of personal safety when you are traveling alone to visit clients.
- **Flexibility.** Each client's home will be different. You will need to adapt to the changes in environment. You will have to learn to work alone with only the client and family to help.
- **Working environment.** In home care, the physical layout of rooms, stairs, lack of equipment, cramped bathrooms, rugs, clutter, and even pets can complicate caregiving.
- **Client's home.** In a client's home, you are a guest. You need to be respectful of the client's property and customs.
- **Clients' comfort.** One of the best things about home care is that it allows clients to stay in the familiar and comfortable surroundings of their own homes.

As an HHA, you will be part of a team of health professionals that includes physicians, nurses, social workers, therapists, and specialists. The client and client's family will interact with the team and are considered part of the team. Everyone involved will work closely together to help clients recover from illnesses or injuries. If full recovery is not possible, the team will help clients do as much as they can for themselves.

The Care Team

Clients will have different needs and problems. Healthcare professionals with different kinds of education and experience will help care for them. Members of the healthcare team may include:

Home Health Aide (HHA). The home health aide performs delegated tasks, such as taking vital signs, and provides routine personal care, such as bathing clients or preparing meals. HHAs spend more time with clients than other care team members do. That is why they act as the "eyes and ears" of the team. Observing and reporting changes in the client's condition or abilities is a very important duty of the HHA.

Case Manager or Supervisor. Usually a registered nurse, a case manager or a supervisor is assigned to each client by the home health agency. The case manager or supervisor, with input from other team members, creates the basic care plan for the client. He or she monitors any changes that are observed and reported by the HHA. The case manager also makes changes in the client care plan when necessary.

Registered Nurse (RN). In a home health agency, a registered nurse coordinates, manages, and provides care. RNs also supervise and train HHAs. They develop the HHA plan of care, or assignments.

Doctor (MD or DO). A doctor's job is to diagnose disease or disability and prescribe treatment. Doctors have graduated from four-year medical schools, which they attended after receiving a bachelor's degree. Many doctors also attend specialized training programs after medical school.

Physical Therapist (PT). The physical therapist administers therapy to muscles, bones, and joints in the form of heat, cold, massage, ultrasound, electricity, and exercise. Goals of physical therapy include improving blood circulation, promoting healing, helping the client regain or maintain mobility, and easing pain.

Occupational Therapist (OT). An occupational therapist helps clients understand and learn to compensate for disabilities. For clients in home care, an occupational therapist may assist in training clients for activities of daily living (ADLs), such as dressing, eating, and bathing.

Speech Language Pathologist (SLP). A speech language pathologist, or speech therapist, identifies and addresses communication disorders. An SLP teaches exercises that help the client improve or overcome speech impediments. An SLP also evaluates a person's ability to swallow food and drink.

Registered Dietitian (RDT). A registered dietitian or nutritionist teaches clients and their families about special diets to improve their health and help them to manage their illness.

Medical Social Worker (MSW). A medical social worker determines clients' needs and helps them get support services, such as counseling, meal services, and financial assistance.

The Care Plan

The client care plan is individualized for each client. It is developed to achieve the specific goals of care. Multiple care plans may be necessary for some clients. In these situations, the supervisor will coordinate the client's overall care. There will be one care plan for the HHA to follow.

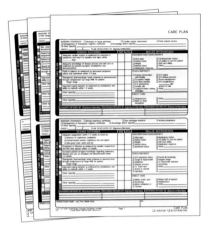

There will be separate care plans for other providers, such as the physical therapist.

The care plan is a guide to help the client attain and maintain the best level of health possible. Activities NOT listed on the HHA care plan should not be performed without permission from the supervisor. The HHA care plan is part of the overall plan of care. It must be followed very carefully.

Care planning should involve input from the client and/or the family, as well as healthcare professionals. Healthcare professionals will assess the client's physical, financial, social, and psychological needs. After the doctor prescribes treatment, the supervisor, nurses, and other care team members create the care plan. Many factors are considered when creating the care plan. They include the client's health and physical condition, diagnosis, treatment, any additional services needed, and the client's home and family.

Care plans must be kept up-to-date as the client's condition changes. Reporting changes and problems to the supervisor is a very important duty of the home health aide. This allows the care team to revise care plans to meet the client's changing needs.

Chain of Command

As a home health aide, you are carrying out instructions given to you by a nurse. The nurse is acting on the instructions of a doctor or other member of the care team. This chain of command guarantees that your clients get proper health care. It also protects you and your employer from liability. Liability is a legal term that means someone can be held responsible for harming someone else. For example, imagine that something you do for a client harms him. However, what you did was in the care plan and was done according to policy and procedure. In this case, you may not be liable, or responsible, for hurting the client. However, if you do something not in the care plan that harms a client, you could be held responsible. That is why it is important to follow instructions in the care plan and for the agency to have a chain of command.

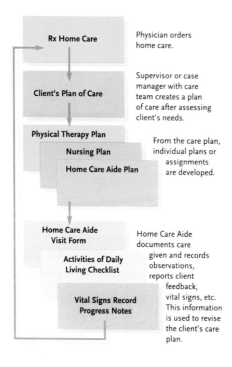

Home health aides must understand what they can and cannot do. This is important so that you do not harm a client or involve yourself or your employer in a lawsuit. Some states certify that a home health aide is qualified to work. However, home health aides are not licensed healthcare providers. Everything you do in your job is assigned to you by a licensed healthcare professional. You do your job under the authority of another person's license. That is why these professionals will show great interest in what you do and how you do it.

Every state grants the right to practice various jobs in health care through licensure. Examples include granting a license to practice nursing, medicine or physical therapy. All members of the healthcare team work under each professional's scope of practice. A scope of practice defines the things you are allowed to do and how to do them correctly.

Policies and Procedures

You will be told where to locate a list of policies and procedures that all staff members are expected to follow. A policy is a course of action that should be taken every time a certain situation occurs. For example, one policy at most agencies is that the care plan must be followed. That means that every time you visit a client, what you do will be determined by the care plan. A procedure is a particular method, or way, of doing something. For example, your agency will have a procedure for reporting information about your clients. The procedure tells you what form you fill out, when and how often to fill it out, and to whom it is given.

Common policies and procedures at home health agencies include the following:

- Keep all information confidential.
- The client's plan of care must be followed.
- HHAs should not do any tasks that are not included in their job description.
- HHAs must report to the supervisor at regular, scheduled times.
- HHAs must report important events or changes in clients and their families.
- Personal problems must not be discussed with the client or the client's family.
- HHAs must be punctual and dependable. Employers expect this of all employees.
- HHAs must meet deadlines for documentation and paperwork.
- HHAs must provide all client care in a pleasant, professional manner.
- HHAs cannot give or receive gifts.

Your employer will have policies and procedures for every client care situation. Though written procedures may seem long and complicated, each step is important.

Professionalism

Professional means having to do with work or a job. The opposite of professional is personal, which refers to parts of your life outside your job. This includes your family, friends, and home life. Professionalism is how you behave when you are on the job. It includes how you dress, the words you use, and the things you talk about. It also includes being on time, finishing your assignments, and reporting to your supervisor. For an HHA, professionalism means participating in care planning, making important observations, and reporting accurately.

Following the policies and procedures of your agency is an important part of professionalism. Clients, coworkers, and supervisors respect employees who behave in a professional way. Professionalism will help you keep your job and may help you earn promotions and raises.

A professional relationship with a client includes:

- maintaining a positive attitude
- being cleanly and neatly dressed and groomed
- arriving on time, doing tasks efficiently, and leaving on time

- finishing assignments
- doing only the tasks assigned
- speaking politely and cheerfully to the client, even if you are not in a good mood
- never cursing or using profanity, even if the client does
- never discussing your personal problems with the client or family
- never giving or accepting gifts
- calling the client "Mr.," "Mrs.," "Ms.," or "Miss," and his or her last name, or by the name he or she prefers
- listening to the client
- always explaining the care you will provide before providing it
- always following care practices, such as handwashing, to protect yourself and the client

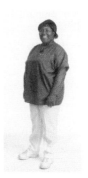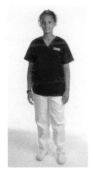

A professional relationship with an employer includes:

- maintaining a positive attitude
- completing assignments efficiently
- consistently following policies and procedures
- documenting and reporting carefully and correctly
- communicating problems with clients or assignments
- reporting anything that keeps you from completing assignments
- asking questions when you do not know or understand something
- taking directions or criticism without getting upset
- always being on time
- participating in education programs offered
- being a positive role model for your agency at all times

Qualities of great HHAs include being compassionate, honest, conscientious, dependable, respectful, unprejudiced, and tolerant.

Legal and Ethical Aspects

Ethics and laws guide our behavior. Ethics are the knowledge of right and wrong. An ethical person has a sense of duty and responsibility toward others. He or she always tries to do what is right. If ethics tell us what we *should* do, laws tell us what we *must* do. Laws are usually based on ethics. Governments establish laws to help people live peacefully together and to ensure order and safety. When someone breaks the law, he or she may be punished by having to pay a fine or spend time in prison.

Ethics and laws are extremely important in health care. They protect people receiving care and guide people giving care. Home health aides and other healthcare providers should be guided by a code of ethics. They must know the laws that apply to their jobs.

Examples of legal and ethical behavior by HHAs include the following:

- being honest at all times
- protecting clients' privacy
- never accepting gifts or tips
- never becoming personally or sexually involved with clients or families
- reporting abuse or suspected abuse of a client
- following the care plan/assignment
- never performing unassigned tasks
- reporting all client observations and incidents
- documenting accurately and on time
- following Standard Precautions

Clients' rights relate to how clients must be treated. They provide an ethical code of conduct for healthcare workers. Home health agencies give clients a list of these rights and review each right with them. Many states require home health agencies to provide their clients with the abuse hotline numbers. And it is a law for HHAs to report suspected cases of abuse.

You can help protect your clients' rights in the following ways:

- Watch for and report to your supervisor any signs of abuse or neglect.
- Involve clients in your planning.
- Always explain a procedure before performing it.
- **Never** abuse a client physically, psychologically, verbally or sexually.
- Respect a client's refusal of care, but report the refusal to your supervisor immediately.

Client Bill of Rights

Home health clients and their formal caregivers have a right to not be discriminated against based on race, color, religion, national origin, age, sex, gender, sexual orientation, or disability. Furthermore, clients and caregivers have a right to mutual respect and dignity, including respect for property. Caregivers are prohibited from accepting personal gifts and borrowing from clients.

CLIENTS HAVE THE RIGHT:

- to have relationships with home health providers that are based on honesty and ethical standards of conduct;

- to be informed of the procedure they can follow to lodge complaints with the home health provider about the care that is, or fails to be, furnished and about a lack of respect for property. [The phone number to report this listed here.]

- to know about the disposition of such complaints;

- to voice their grievances without fear of discrimination or reprisal for having done so; and

- to be advised of the telephone number and hours of operation of the state's home care hotline which receives questions and complaints about local home care agencies, including complaints about implementation of advance directive requirements. [Hours and phone number listed here.]

CLIENTS HAVE THE RIGHT:

- to be notified in advance about the care that is to be furnished, the types (disciplines) of the caregivers who will furnish the care, and the frequency of the visits that are proposed to be furnished;

- to be advised of any change in the plan of care before the change is made;

- to participate in the planning of the care and in planning changes in the care, and to be advised that they have the right to do so;

- to be informed in writing of rights under state law to make decisions concerning medical care, including the right to accept or refuse treatment and the right to formulate advance directives;

- to be notified of the expected outcomes of care and any obstacles or barriers to treatment*

- to be informed in writing of policies and procedures for implementing advance directives, including any limitations if the provider cannot implement an advance directive on the basis of conscience;

- to have health care providers comply with advance directives in accordance with state law requirements;

- to receive care without condition on, or discrimination based on, the execution of advance directives; and

- to refuse services without fear of reprisal or discrimination.

* The home care provider or the client's physician may be forced to refer the client to another source of care if the client's refusal to comply with the plan of care threatens to compromise the provider's commitment to quality care.

CLIENTS HAVE THE RIGHT:

- to confidentiality of the medical record as well as information about their health, social, and financial circumstances and about what takes place in the home; and

- to expect the home care provider to release information only as required by law or authorized by the client and to be informed of procedures for disclosure.

CLIENTS HAVE THE RIGHT:

- to be informed of the extent to which payment may be expected from Medicare, Medicaid, or any other payer known to the home care provider;

- to be informed of the charges that will not be covered by Medicare;

- to be informed of the charges for which the client may be liable;

Continues on next page

- to receive this information, orally and in writing, before care is initiated and within 30 calendar days of the date the home care provider becomes aware of any changes; and

- to have access, upon request, to all bills for service the client has received regardless of whether the bills are paid out-of-pocket or by another party.

CLIENTS HAVE THE RIGHT:

- to receive care of the highest quality;

- in general, to be admitted by a home health provider only if it has the resources needed to provide the care safely and at the required level of intensity, as determined by a professional assessment; a provider with less than optimal resources may nevertheless admit the client if a more appropriate provider is not available, but only after fully informing the client of the provider's limitations and the lack of suitable alternative arrangements; and

- to be told what to do in the case of an emergency.

THE HOME HEALTH PROVIDER SHALL ASSURE THAT:

- all medically related home care is provided in accordance with physicians' orders and that a plan of care specifies the services and their frequency and duration; and

- all medically related personal care is provided by an appropriately trained home health aide who is supervised by a nurse or other qualified home care professional.

CLIENTS HAVE THE RESPONSIBILITY:

- to notify the provider of changes in their condition (e.g., hospitalization, changes in the plan of care, symptoms to be reported);

- to follow the plan of care;

- to notify the provider if the visit schedule needs to be changed;

- to inform providers of the existence of any changes made to advance directives;

- to advise the provider of any problems or dissatisfaction with the services provided;

- to provide a safe environment for care to be provided; and

- to carry out mutually-agreed-upon responsibilities.

To satisfy the Medicare certification requirements, the Centers for Medicare & Medicaid Services (CMS) requires that agencies:

1. Give a copy of the Bill of Rights to each client in the course of the admission process.

2. Explain the Bill of Rights to the client and document that this has been done.

Agencies may have clients sign a copy of the client's Bill of Rights to acknowledge receipt.

- Tell your supervisor if a client has questions about the goals of care or the care plan.

- Be truthful when documenting care.

- Do not talk or gossip about a client.

- Knock and ask permission before entering a client's room.

- Do not open a client's mail or look through his belongings.

- Do not accept gifts or money from a client.

- Respect your clients' property.
- Report observations regarding a client's condition or care.

ABUSE AND NEGLECT: OBSERVING AND REPORTING

- Physical abuse—unexplained injuries including burns, bruises, and bone injuries
- Emotional abuse—complaints of anxiety, signs of stress, withdrawal from others, or fear of family members, friends, or authority figures
- Neglect—signs of lack of care when HHA is not present, such as incontinence briefs not changed or lack of food in the house

Negligence means the failure to provide the proper care for a client which results in unintended injury. Some examples of negligence include:

- Not noticing that your client's dentures do not fit properly. Therefore, he is not eating well and becomes malnourished.
- Not replacing a hearing aid battery. Your client does not hear the smoke alarm, but is rescued by a neighbor who does hear it.
- Not observing that your client's eyesight is getting worse. Corrective measures are not taken, and she falls and is injured.

To respect confidentiality means to keep private things private. You will learn confidential (private) information about your clients. You may learn about a client's state of health, finances, and personal relationships. Ethically and legally, you must protect the confidentiality of this information. This means you should not tell anyone other than members of the healthcare team anything about your clients.

Congress passed the Health Insurance Portability and Accountability Act (HIPAA) in 1996. It was further defined and revised in 2001 and 2002. One of the reasons this law was passed is to help keep health information private and secure. All healthcare organizations must take special steps to protect health information. They and their employees can be fined and/or imprisoned if they do not follow special rules to protect privacy. This applies to all healthcare providers, including doctors, nurses, home health aides, and any members of the care team.

Under this law a person's health information must be kept private. It is called protected health information (PHI). Examples of PHI include name, address, telephone number, social security number, e-mail address, and medical record number. Only people who must have information to provide care or to process records should know a person's private health information. They must make sure they protect the information so it does not become known or used by anyone else. It must be kept confidential.

HHAs cannot give any information about a client to anyone who is not directly involved in the client's care unless the client gives official consent or unless the law requires it. For example, if a neighbor asks you how your client is doing, you should reply, "I'm sorry but I cannot share that information. It's confidential." That is the correct response to anyone who does not have a legal reason to know about the client.

All healthcare workers must comply with HIPAA regulations, no matter where they are or what they are doing. There are serious penalties for violating these regulations. Penalties differ depending upon the violation and can include fines and prison sentences.

Maintaining confidentiality is a legal and ethical obligation. It is part of respecting your clients and their rights. Your clients have to trust you. Talking about them betrays this trust. Discussing a client's care or personal affairs with anyone other than your supervisor or another member of the healthcare team violates the law.

II
Foundation of Client Care

4. Communication

Communication is the process by which we exchange information with others. It is a process of sending and receiving messages. People communicate by using signs and symbols, such as words, drawings, and pictures. They also communicate by their behavior.

Effective communication is a critical part of your job. HHAs must communicate with supervisors, members of the care team, clients, and family members. A client's health depends on how well you communicate your observations and concerns to your supervisor. You will also need to be able to communicate clearly and respectfully in stressful or confusing situations.

Clients may sometimes display combative, meaning violent or hostile, behavior. Such behavior may include hitting, pushing, kicking, or verbal attacks. This behavior may be the result of disease affecting the brain. It may also be an expression of frustration. Or it may just be part of someone's personality. In general, combative behavior is not a reaction to you. Do not take it personally.

Always report combative behavior to your supervisor and document it. Even if you do not find the behavior upsetting, the care team needs to be aware of it. Some ways of coping with combative behavior include the following:

- Block physical blows or step out of the way, but never hit back.
- Leave the client alone if you can safely do so.
- Do not respond to verbal attacks.
- Consider what provoked the client.
- Report inappropriate behavior to your supervisor.

Barriers to Communication

Communication can be blocked or disrupted in many ways. Following are some barriers and ways to avoid them:

- Client does not hear you, does not hear correctly, or does not understand. Stand directly facing the client. Speak more slowly than you do with family and friends. Speak clearly, in a pleasant voice.

- Client is difficult to understand. Be patient and take time to listen. Ask client to repeat or explain. Try to rephrase the message in your own words to make sure you have understood.

- Message uses words receiver does not understand. Do not use medical terminology with clients. Speak in simple, everyday words. Ask what a word means if you are not sure.

- Using slang confuses the message. Avoid using slang words and expressions that are unprofessional and may not be understood.

- Using clichés makes your message meaningless. Clichés are phrases that are used over and over again and don't really mean anything.

- Asking "why" makes the client defensive. Avoid asking "why" when a client makes a statement.

- Giving advice is inappropriate. Do not offer your personal opinion or give advice.

- Nonverbal communication changes the message. Be aware of your body language and gestures when you are speaking.

- Client may speak a different language. You may need to use pictures or gestures to communicate.

Oral Reports

Ask for more. When clients report symptoms, events, or feelings, have them repeat what they have said and ask them for more information. Avoid asking questions that can be easily answered with a simple "yes" or "no" response. Instead ask questions that encourage the client to offer more descriptive information. For example, asking the client, "Did you sleep well last night?" could easily be answered "yes" or "no." However, asking the client, "Tell me about your night and how you slept," is more likely to encourage the client to offer facts and details.

HHAs must be able to make brief and accurate oral and written presentations to clients and staff. Reports of a client's status are used in two ways. The first is to report something your supervisor needs to know about immediately. Signs and symptoms that should be reported will be discussed throughout this book. In addition, anything that endangers your client should be reported immediately. Examples include the following:

- falls
- chest pain
- severe headache
- difficulty breathing
- abnormal pulse, respiration, or blood pressure
- change in client's mental status
- sudden weakness or loss of mobility
- high fever
- loss of consciousness
- change in level of consciousness
- bleeding
- change in client's condition
- bruises, abrasions, or other signs of possible abuse

Another way to use oral reports is to discuss your experiences with a client or family member and your observations of the client's condition and care. Even for oral reports, write notes so you do not forget any details. You will also have to make a written report later, so you'll need to be able to recall all the facts accurately. Following an oral report, document when, why, about what, and to whom an oral report was given.

Sometimes your supervisor or another member of the care team will give you a brief oral report on one of your clients. Listen carefully and take notes if you need to. Ask about anything you do not understand. At the end of the conversation, restate what you have been told to make sure you understand.

In order to report accurately, you must observe your clients, their families, and their homes. To observe accurately, use as many senses as possible to gather information. Some examples follow.

- **Sight.** Look for changes in client's appearance. These include rashes, redness, paleness, swelling, discharge, weakness, sunken eyes, and posture or gait (walking) changes. Look for changes in the home. Does the home appear disorganized or dirty? Is food needed? Do safety hazards exist?

- **Hearing.** Listen to what the client tells you about his or her condition, family, or needs. Is the client speaking clearly and making sense? Does the client show emotions such as anger, frustration, or sadness? Is breathing normal? Does client wheeze, gasp, or cough? Listen to family members' observations about the client's needs or condition. Is the area calm and quiet enough for your client to rest as needed?

- **Touch.** Does your client's skin feel hot or cool, moist or dry? Is pulse rate normal? Use your sense of touch to test the bath water and the home's heating or cooling system.

- **Smell.** Do you notice odor from the client's body? Odors could suggest inadequate bathing, infections, or incontinence. Breath odor could suggest use of alcohol or tobacco, indigestion, or poor oral care. Odors in the home may suggest housecleaning or repairs are needed. Food odors could indicate spoilage.

Using all your senses will allow you to make the most complete report of a client's situation.

Documentation

Maintaining current documentation means keeping a record of everything you do and observe during a client visit. You and your agency maintain current documentation for these reasons:

1 It is the only way to guarantee clear and complete communication between all the members of the care team.

2 Documentation is a legal record of every part of a client's treatment. It is proof that a visit was actually made. Medical charts can be used in court as legal evidence.

3 Documentation protects you and your employer from liability by proving what you did on every visit with your client.

4 Documentation on the client's visit form provides an up-to-date record of each of your clients' status and care.

Visit records, progress notes, or clinical notes are the notes you make each time you visit a client. These notes serve as a record of your visit and the care you provided. Visit records also document observations of the client's condition, change, or progress (improvement). When writing visit records, observe these rules:

1 Write your notes immediately after the visit. This helps you remember important details. Always wait to document until after you have completed care. Never record any care before it is done.

2 Think about what you want to say before writing. This will help you present your thoughts as briefly and as clearly as possible.

3 Write the facts, not your opinions. For example, "Client has lost 2 lb. Did not finish lunch," reports facts. It is more useful than "Client is thin and won't eat." When reporting something a client or family member told you, put the words in quotation marks (" "). Document the tasks that you performed, assisted with, or observed.

4 Write as neatly as you can. Use black ink.

5 If you make a mistake, draw one line through it. Write the correct word or words. Put your initials and the date. Never erase something you have written. Never use correction fluid.

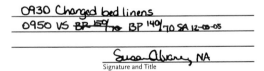

6 Sign your full name, write your title (Home Health Aide, Aide, or HHA). Write the date after each day's visit notes.

7 Document as specified in the care plan. Some agencies have a "check-off" sheet for documenting care. It is also called an ADL (activities of daily living) sheet.

Incident reports must be completed when an accident or other significant event occurs during a visit. Report the incident as soon as possible. Report it before leaving the client's home. Always check with your supervisor before completing the report. Every home health agency has its own policies and procedures for incident reporting.

In general, file a report when any of the following incidents occur:

• your client falls

• you or a client break or damage something

• your client or a family member makes a request that is out of your scope of practice or not on your assignment

• your client or a family member makes sexual advances or remarks

- anything happens that makes you feel uncomfortable, threatened, or unsafe

- you get injured on the job

- you are exposed to blood or body fluids

An incident report documents events that happen in the home and protects you. It provides a written record of anything that happens and describes your part in it. Most agencies use incident reports in place of writing up the accident on the visit form. You may be asked to document that you completed an incident report.

Telephone Communication

You will use the telephone to communicate with your supervisor. Always ask permission before using a client's phone. You may also need to answer the phone for your clients and know how to take messages.

When making a call, follow these steps:

1 Always identify yourself before asking to speak to someone. Never ask "Who is this?" when someone answers your call.

2 After you have identified yourself, ask for the person with whom you need to speak.

3 If the person you are calling is available, identify yourself again. State why you are calling. Plan your call before you pick up the phone. This will help you be as efficient as possible.

4 If the person is not available, ask if you can leave a message. Always leave a message, even if it is only to say you called. The message shows that you were trying to reach someone.

5 Leave a brief and clear message. Do not give more information than necessary.

6 Thank the person who takes the message for you. Always be polite over the telephone, as you would in person.

5. Infection Control

This section provides a brief review of infection control, Standard Precautions, and Transmission-Based, or Isolation, Precautions. It is intended only as a brief review of concepts and skills with which you may already be familiar.

Preventing the spread of infection is as important in the home as in any other healthcare setting. The difference is that in the home a great responsibility rests on the caregiver. There is no facility present to supply the proper equipment or enforce policies or procedures. Be familiar with the infection control practices of your agency. This includes all policies and procedures affecting your day-to-day tasks. There are no high faucets or deep sinks with special liquid soap and paper towel dispensers in most homes. You will be expected to adapt to what is actually available for your use. Therefore, assess the home for available infection control resources first. Plan how you will follow the appropriate standards of care. This includes the proper precautions to prevent and control infection.

Home Care Bag

In some situations, it may be a good idea for the HHA to carry a "home care bag." This bag can contain needed supplies, such as gloves, special handwashing wipes or soaps, paper towels, alcohol wipes, and a personal protective equipment (PPE) kit for emergencies. This special bag, such as a small duffel bag, should be used in place of a purse. A purse can become contaminated when carried from house to house. This bag should not be placed on the floor or on the client's bed or table. It should be placed on clean pieces of newspaper which the family can provide. Put it in an area close to where the client's care will be given. Designate this area as the "home care corner." This is an excellent spot to keep any other supplies caregivers might need as they care for the client. These include gloves, care plans, education materials, and dressings and tape.

Spread of Infection

Asepsis means no pathogens are present. It refers to the clean conditions you want to create in the home. Preventing the spread of infection is important. To know how to do this, you must first know how infection is spread. The chain of infection describes how disease is transmitted from one being to another. Definitions and examples of the six links in the chain of infection are:

Link 1: The **causative agent** is a pathogen or microorganism that causes disease. Examples include bacteria, viruses, fungi, and protozoa.

Link 2: A **reservoir** is a place where the pathogen lives and grows. Examples include the lungs, blood, and large intestine.

Link 3: The **portal of exit** is any body opening on an infected person that allows pathogens to leave, such as the nose, mouth, eyes, or a cut in skin.

Link 4: The **mode of transmission** describes how the pathogen travels from one person to the next person. Transmission can happen through the air or through direct contact or indirect contact.

Link 5: The **portal of entry** is any body opening on an uninfected person that allows pathogens to enter. This can occur through the nose, mouth, eyes, other mucous membranes, a cut in the skin, or dry/cracked skin.

Link 6: A **susceptible host** is an uninfected person who could get sick. Examples include all healthcare workers and anyone in their care who is not already infected with that particular disease.

If one of the links in the chain of infection is broken, then the spread of infection is stopped.

Standard Precautions

The Centers for Disease Control and Prevention (CDC) is a federal government agency that issues guidelines to protect and improve health. The CDC tries to control and prevent disease. In 1996, the CDC recommended a new infection control system to reduce the risk of contracting infectious diseases. In 2004, the CDC proposed some changes to this system.

There are two levels of precautions within the infection control system. They are Standard Precautions and Transmission-Based, or Isolation, Precautions. In the 2004 proposed guidelines the CDC suggests that the term "Expanded Precautions" be used instead of "Transmission-Based Precautions."

Following Standard Precautions means treating all blood, body fluids, non-intact skin (like abrasions, pimples, or open sores), and mucous membranes (lining of mouth, nose, eyes, rectum, or genitals) as if they were infected. Standard Precautions are simple to remember because they include everything except sweat. Under Standard Precautions, "body fluids" include saliva, sputum (mucus coughed up), urine, feces, semen, vaginal secretions, and pus or other wound drainage.

Standard Precautions must be practiced on every single person in your care. This is the only safe way of doing your job. You cannot tell by looking at your residents or their charts if they have an infectious disease such as HIV, hepatitis, or influenza.

Standard Precautions include the measures below:

- Wear gloves if you may come into contact with: blood; body fluids or secretions; broken skin (abrasions, acne, cuts, stitches or staples); or mucous membranes (linings of the mouth, nose, eyes, vagina, rectum, and penis). Such situations include mouth care; bathroom assistance; perineal care; helping with a bedpan or urinal; ostomy care; cleaning up spills; cleaning basins, urinals, bedpans, and other containers that have held body fluids; and disposing of wastes.

- Wash your hands before putting on gloves. Wash them immediately after removing your gloves. Be careful not to touch clean objects with your used gloves.

- Remove gloves immediately when finished with a procedure.

- Immediately wash all skin surfaces that have been contaminated with blood and body fluids.

- Wear a disposable gown if you may come into contact with blood or body fluids.

- Wear a mask and protective goggles if you may come into contact with splashing or spraying blood or body fluids.

- Wear gloves and use caution when handling razor blades, needles, and other sharps. Sharps are needles or other sharp objects. Discard them carefully in a puncture-resistant biohazard container.

- Never attempt to cap needles or sharps. Dispose of them in an approved container.

- Avoid nicks and cuts when shaving clients.

- Carefully bag all contaminated supplies. Dispose of them according to your agency's policy.

- Clearly label body fluids that are saved for a specimen with the client's name and a biohazard label. Keep them in a container with a lid.

- Dispose of contaminated wastes according to your agency's policy.

Handwashing

Washing your hands is the single most important thing you can do to prevent the spread of disease. The CDC has defined hand hygiene as handwashing with either plain or antiseptic soap and water and using alcohol-based hand rubs. Alcohol-based hand rubs include gels, rinses, and foams. They do not require the use of water.

Alcohol-based hand rubs have proven effective in reducing bacteria on the skin. However, they are not a substitute for proper handwashing. Always use soap and water for visibly soiled hands. It is important to wash your hands often. Once they are clean, alcohol-based products can be used in addition to handwashing. Use hand lotion to prevent dry, cracked skin.

If you wear rings, consider removing them while working. Rings may increase the risk of contamination. Keep fingernails short and clean. Do not wear false nails. False nails increase the risk of contamination.

The following are three possible problem areas for the aide to assess in the home regarding handwashing:

- Where will you wash your hands? Does the bathroom sink or the kitchen sink have a higher faucet and plenty of hot water?

- What soap will you use? Does the family have an anti-bacterial soap dispenser at that sink? Never use the family's bar of soap for yourself.

- How will you dry your hands? Are there paper towels and a wastebasket close by? Never use the family's bathroom or kitchen towels for yourself or your client.

You should wash your hands:

- when arriving at a client's home
- before and after touching a client
- before and after making meals or working in the kitchen
- before and after you eat
- before feeding a client
- after using the bathroom
- after touching any item used by or for a client
- before leaving a client's home
- before reaching into the clean area of your supply bag
- before putting on gloves
- after removing gloves or any type of personal protection equipment (PPE)
- after touching a surface that may be contaminated with any body fluid

Washing hands

Equipment: bar or liquid soap provided by your employer, paper
towels

1   Turn on water at sink. Keep your
clothes dry, because moisture
breeds bacteria.

2   Angle your arms down, holding
your hands lower than your
elbows. This prevents water from
running up your arm. Wet hands
and wrists thoroughly.

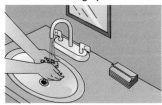

3   Use a generous amount of soap.
Rub hands together and fingers
between each other to create a
lather. Lather all surfaces of fingers and hands, including above
the wrists, producing friction for at
least 10 seconds. Friction helps
clean.

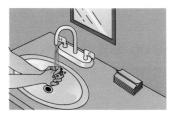

4   Clean your nails by pushing soap
under your fingernails and cuticles
with a brush or by rubbing them
in the palm of your hand.

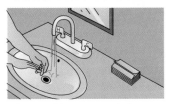

5   Being careful not to touch the
sink, rinse thoroughly under running water. Rinse from just above
the wrists down to fingertips. Do
not run water over unwashed arm
down to clean hands.

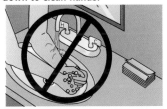

6   Using a clean paper towel, dry
from tips of fingers up to clean
wrists. Do not wipe towel on
unwashed forearms and then wipe
clean hands. Dispose of towel
without touching waste container.
If your hands ever touch the sink
or waste container, start over.

7   Use a dry, clean paper towel to
turn off the faucet without contaminating your hands. Properly
discard towel.

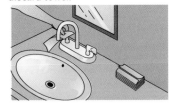

Always wear gloves when there is a chance you might come into contact
with body fluids, open wounds, or mucous membranes. This includes:

• anytime you might touch blood or any body fluid, including vomit,
urine, feces, or saliva

• performing or assisting with mouth care or care of any mucous
membrane

- performing or assisting with care of the perineal (payr-i-NEE-al) area (the area between and including the anus and the genitals)

- performing personal care on a client whose skin is broken by abrasions, cuts, rash, acne, pimples, or boils

- assisting with a client's personal care when you have open sores or cuts on your hands

- shaving a client

- disposing of soiled bed linens, gowns, dressings, and pads

GUIDELINES: WEARING GLOVES

- Cover any cuts or sores on your hands with bandages or gauze and then put on gloves.

- Disposable gloves are to be worn only once. They may not be washed or disinfected for reuse. Change gloves right before contact with mucous membranes or broken skin, or if gloves are soiled, torn, or damaged. Wash your hands before putting on fresh gloves.

Some people are allergic to the latex used in certain gloves. If you notice a reaction, contact your supervisor immediately. Your employer will provide you with a kind of glove you can wear.

Putting on gloves

1   Wash your hands.

2   If you are right-handed, slide one glove on your left hand (reverse if left-handed).

3   With gloved hand, take second glove and slide the other hand into the glove.

4   Interlace fingers to smooth out folds and create a comfortable fit.

5   Carefully look for tears, holes, or discolored spots. Replace the glove if necessary.

6   If wearing a gown, pull the cuff of the gloves over the sleeve of the gown.

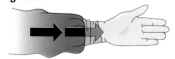

Remove gloves promptly after use and before caring for another client. Wash your hands. Remove your gloves before touching non-contaminated items or surfaces. You are wearing gloves to protect your skin from contamination. After giving care, your gloves are contaminated. If you open a door with the gloved hand, the doorknob is contaminated. Later, when you open the door with an ungloved hand, you will be infected. It is a common mistake to contaminate the room around you. Do not do this. Before touching surfaces, remove gloves. Wash your hands. Put on new gloves if needed.

Taking off gloves

1 Touching only the outside of one glove, pull the first glove off by pulling down from the cuff.

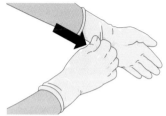
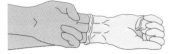

remaining glove, being careful not to touch any part of the outside.

4 Pull down, turning this glove inside out and over the first glove as you remove it.

2 As the glove comes off your hand it should be turned inside out.

5 You should be holding one glove from its clean inner side and the other glove should be inside it.

3 With the fingertips of your gloved hand hold the glove you just removed. With your ungloved hand, reach two fingers *inside* the

6 Drop both gloves into the proper container.

7 Wash your hands.

Personal Protective Equipment (PPE)

In addition to gloves, PPE includes gowns, masks, and eye shields (goggles). Your employer will provide you with PPE as necessary for your client assignments. The guidelines for wearing PPE are the same as for gloves. You should wear PPE if there is a chance you could come into contact with body fluids, mucous membranes, or open wounds. Masks and eye shields are worn when splashing of body fluids or blood could occur. Masks should also be worn when caring for clients with respiratory illnesses.

Putting on a gown

1 Wash your hands.

2 Open gown. Hold out in front of you and allow gown to open. Do not shake it. Slip your arms into the sleeves and pull the gown on.

3 Tie the neck ties into a bow so they can be easily untied later.

4 Reaching behind you, pull the gown until it completely covers your clothes. Tie the back ties.

5 Remember, use gown only once and then remove and discard it. When removing a gown, roll the

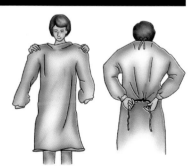

dirty side in and away from the body. If your gown ever becomes wet or soiled, remove it. Check your clothing, and put on a new gown. The Occupational Safety and Health Administration (OSHA) requires non-permeable gowns, that is, gowns that liquids cannot penetrate, when working in a bloody situation.

6 Put on gloves after putting on gown.

Putting on a mask and goggles

1 Wash your hands.

2 Pick up mask by the top strings or the elastic strap. Be careful not to touch the mask where it touches your face. Do not wear the same mask from one client to another.

3 Adjust the mask over your nose and mouth. Tie top strings first, then bottom strings. Masks must always be dry or they must be replaced. Never wear a mask hanging from only the bottom ties.

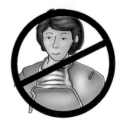

4 Put on the goggles.

5 Put on gloves after putting on mask and goggles.

Special Precautions

Spills in the home, especially those involving blood, body fluids, or glass, can pose a serious risk of infection. Hospitals and long-term care settings have special types of flooring and specific commercial solutions they use for spills. In the home, such products may not be available. More carpet and rugs may create a challenge for the aide to clean. When you are caring for a client who has a known infection, it is advisable to ask the family to purchase special anti-bacterial cleaners. Reading the label carefully is important because certain precautions may need to be taken with their use. For example, they may contain bleach that could take the color out of a carpet as well as removing the stain or spill.

GUIDELINES: CLEANING SPILLS
INVOLVING BLOOD, BODY FLUIDS, OR GLASS

- When blood or body fluids are spilled, put on gloves before starting to clean up the spill. In some cases, industrial strength gloves are best because they will not tear if you are also handling glass.

- When glass has been broken, do not pick up any pieces, no matter how large, with your hands. Use a dustpan and broom or other tools.

- If blood or body fluids are spilled on a hard surface such as a linoleum floor or countertop, clean immediately using a solution of one part household bleach to ten parts water. You can mix the solution in a bucket, and, with gloves on, wipe up the spill with rags or paper towels dipped in the solution. Or, mix the solution in a plastic spray bottle and spray the spill before wiping.

- If blood or body fluids are spilled on fabrics such as carpets, bedding, or clothes, do not use bleach to clean the spill. Commercial disinfectants that do not contain bleach are available. Use gloves to load soiled bedding or clothes into the washing machine and add color-safe bleach to the washer with the laundry detergent.

- Waste containing broken glass, blood, or body fluids should be properly bagged. Put the waste in one trash bag and close it properly. Then put the first bag inside a second, clean trash bag and close it. This is called double-bagging. Waste containing blood or body fluids may need to be placed in a special biohazard waste bag and disposed of separately from household trash. Follow your agency's policy.

Infectious Disease Precautions

In 1996, the CDC set forth a second level of precautions beyond the Standard Precautions. These guidelines were for persons who are infected or may be infected with diseases. They were known as Transmission-Based, or Isolation, Precautions. If approved, the new name for these precautions will be "Expanded Precautions."

GUIDELINES: INFECTIOUS DISEASES

- Always follow Standard Precautions.

- Wash your hands frequently, especially after client care.

- Use gloves, gowns, masks, and eye shields when needed.

- Follow isolation procedures described in the assignment sheet for each client.

- Handle laundry, personal items, and waste carefully.

There are several categories of Transmission-Based Precautions. The category used depends on the disease and how it spreads. They may also be used in combination for diseases that have multiple routes of transmission. Transmission-Based Precautions are always used **in addition** to Standard Precautions.

Airborne Precautions

Used for diseases that are transmitted through the air after being expelled. The pathogens are so small that they can attach to moisture in the air. They remain floating for some time. For certain care you will be required to wear a N95 mask or a HEPA respirator to avoid infection. Airborne diseases include tuberculosis, measles, and chicken pox.

Droplet Precautions

Used when the disease-causing microorganism does not remain in the air. These pathogens usually travel only short distances after being expelled. Droplets normally do not travel more than three feet. Droplets can be created by coughing, sneezing, talking, laughing, or suctioning. Droplet Precautions include wearing a face mask during care and restricting visits from uninfected people. Cover your nose and mouth with a tissue when you sneeze or cough. Ask clients, family, and others to do the same. If you sneeze on your hands, wash them promptly. An example of a droplet disease is the mumps.

Contact Precautions

Used when the client is at risk of transmitting a microorganism by touching an infected object or person. Examples include bacteria that could infect an open skin wound or infection. Lice, scabies (a skin disease that causes itching), and conjunctivitis (pink eye) are also examples. Transmission can occur during transfers or bathing. Contact Precautions include PPE and client isolation. They require washing hands with antimicrobial soap. They also require not touching contaminated surfaces with ungloved hands or uninfected surfaces with contaminated gloves.

Two important points to remember are:

1 When they are indicated, Transmission-Based Precautions are always used IN ADDITION to Standard Precautions.

2 The client must be reassured that it is the disease, not the person, that is being isolated. Talk with your client. Explain why these steps are being taken.

Several state and federal government agencies have guidelines and laws concerning infection control. OSHA requires employers to provide for the safety of their employees through rules and suggested guidelines. The Centers for Disease Control issues guidelines for healthcare workers to follow on the job. Some of the infection control requirements for you and your employer are listed below.

Employer's responsibilities for infection control include the following:

- Establish infection control procedures and an exposure control plan to protect workers.

- Provide continuing in-service education on infection control, including bloodborne and airborne pathogens.
- Have written procedures to follow should an exposure occur, including medical treatment and plans to prevent similar exposures.
- Provide PPE for employees to use and train them on when and how to properly use it.
- Provide free hepatitis B vaccinations for all "at-risk employees." As a home health aide, you are considered at-risk.

Employee's responsibilities for infection control include the following:

- Follow Standard Precautions.
- Follow all agency policies and procedures.
- Follow client care plans and assignments.
- Use provided PPE as indicated or appropriate.
- Take advantage of the free hepatitis B vaccination.
- Immediately report any exposure you have to infection, blood, or body fluids.
- Participate in annual education programs covering infection control.

6. Safety and Body Mechanics

Principles of Body Mechanics

Body mechanics is the way the parts of the body work together whenever you move. Good body mechanics can save energy, prevent injury, and help you push, pull, and lift objects or people.

The ABC's of good body mechanics are:

Alignment. When standing, sitting, or lying down, you should try to have your body in alignment. This means that the two sides of the body are mirror images of each other, with body parts lined up naturally. Maintain correct body alignment when lifting or carrying an object by keeping the object close to your body. Point your feet and body in the direction you are moving. Avoid twisting at the waist.

Base of support. The base of support is the foundation that supports an object. The feet are the body's base of support. The wider your support, the more stable you are. Standing with legs apart allows for a greater base of support. It is more stable than standing with the feet close together.

Center of gravity. The center of gravity in your body is the point where the most weight is concentrated. This point will depend on the position the body is in. When you stand, your weight is centered in your pelvis. A low center of gravity gives a more stable base of support. Bending your knees when lifting an object lowers your pelvis and, therefore, lowers your center of gravity. This gives you more stability and makes you less likely to fall or strain the working muscles.

Some common examples of applying body mechanics include the following:

Lifting a heavy object from the floor. Spread your feet shoulder-width apart and bend your knees. Using the strong, large muscles in your thighs, upper arms, and shoulders, lift the object. Pull it close to your body, to a point level with your pelvis. By doing this you are keeping the object close to your center of gravity and base of support. When you stand up, push with your strong hip and thigh muscles to raise your body and the object together.

Do not twist when you are moving an object. Always face the object or person you are moving. Pivot your feet instead of twisting at the waist.

Helping a client sit up, stand up, or walk. Whenever you need to support a client's weight, protect yourself by assuming a good stance. Place your feet about 12 inches or hip-width apart, one foot in front of the other, with your knees bent. Your upper body should stay upright and in alignment.

If the client starts to fall, you will be in a good position to help support him or her. Never try to catch a falling client. If a client falls, assist him or her to the floor. If you try to reverse a fall in progress, you will probably injure yourself and/or the client.

Bend your knees to lower yourself, rather than bending from the waist. Any time a task requires bending, use a good stance. This allows you to use the big muscles in your legs and hips rather than straining the smaller muscles in your back.

If you are making an adjustable bed, adjust the height to working level, usually waist high. If you are making a regular bed, put one knee on the bed, lean, or even kneel to support yourself at working level. Avoid bending at the waist.

Keep the following tips in mind to avoid strain and injury:

- Use both arms and hands when lifting, pulling, pushing, or carrying objects.

- Hold objects close to you when you are lifting or carrying them.

- Push, slide, or pull objects rather than lifting them.

- Avoid bending and reaching as much as possible. Move or position furniture so that you do not have to bend or reach.

- Avoid twisting at the waist. Instead, turn your whole body. Your feet should point toward what you are lifting.

- When moving a client, let him know what you will do so he can help if possible. Count to three and lift or move on three so everyone moves together.

- Report to your supervisor if your assignments include tasks you feel you cannot safely perform.

- Never attempt to lift an object or a client that you feel you cannot handle.

Following are several strategies that can help you apply good body mechanics in the home:

- **Have the right tools for a job.** For example, if you cannot reach an object on a high shelf, use a step stool rather than climbing on a counter or straining to reach.

- **Have footrests and pillows available.** For example, tasks that require standing for long periods can be more comfortable if you rest one foot on a footrest. This position flexes the muscles in the lower back and keeps the spine in alignment.

- **When sitting, using a footrest allows for a more comfortable leg position.** Crossing the legs disrupts alignment. It should be avoided. Using pillows can make any chair more comfortable. Use pillows behind the back to keep the back straight.

- **Keep tools, supplies, and clutter off the floor.** Keep frequently-used items on shelves or counters where they can be easily reached without lifting. Keeping things organized will also help you find what you need without straining.

- **Sit when you can.** Whenever you can sit to do a job, do so. Chopping vegetables, folding clothes, and other tasks can be done easily while sitting. For jobs like scouring the bathtub, kneel or use a low stool. Avoid bending at the waist.

- **Use gait or transfer belts when assisting clients with ambulation or transfers.** In Section IV you will learn correct procedures for safely assisting clients with ambulation and transfers.

Accident Prevention

Falls. Falls are among the most common home accidents. Falls can be caused by an unsafe environment or by loss of abilities. Falls are particularly common among the elderly. Older people are often more seriously injured by falls because their bones are more fragile.

Factors that raise the risk of falls include:

- clutter
- throw rugs
- exposed electrical cords
- slippery floors
- uneven floors or stairs
- poor lighting

Personal conditions that raise the risk of falls include medications, loss of vision, gait or balance disturbances, weakness, paralysis or paresis (pa-REE-sis, or partial paralysis), and disorientation. Disorientation means confusion about time or place.

Follow these guidelines to guard against falls:

- Clear all walkways of clutter, throw rugs, and cords.
- Avoid waxing floors, and use non-skid mats or carpeting where appropriate.
- Immediately clean up spills on the floor.
- Mark uneven flooring or stairs with red tape to indicate a hazard.
- Improve lighting where necessary.

Burns/Scalds. Burns can be caused by stoves and electrical appliances, hot water or liquids, or heating devices. Small children, older adults, or people with loss of sensation due to paralysis are at greatest risk of burns. Scalds are burns caused by hot liquids. It takes five seconds or less for a serious burn to occur when the temperature of liquid is 140°F. Coffee, tea, and other hot drinks are usually served at 160°F to 180°F. Follow these guidelines to guard against burns and scalds:

- Roll up sleeves and avoid loose clothing when working at the stove.
- Check that the stove and appliances are off when you leave.
- Suggest that the hot water heater be set lower than normal. It should be set at 120°F to 130°F to avoid burns from scalding tap water.
- Always check water temperature with water thermometer or on wrist before using.
- Check temperatures of liquids on your wrist before serving.
- Keep space heaters away from clients' beds, chairs, and draperies. Never allow space heaters to be used in the bathroom.
- Report frayed electrical cords or unsafe-looking appliances immediately. Do not use these appliances.
- Let clients know you are about to pour or set down a hot liquid.
- Pour hot drinks away from clients.
- Keep hot drinks and liquids away from edges of tables. Put a lid on them.
- Make sure clients are sitting down before serving hot drinks.

Poisoning. Homes contain many harmful substances that should not be swallowed. These include cleaning products, paints, medicines, toiletries, and glues. Follow these guidelines to guard against poisoning:

- Lock harmful products away from confused clients, clients with limited vision, and children.
- Have the number for the Poison Control Center posted by the telephone.

Cuts. Cuts typically occur in the kitchen or bathroom. Follow these guidelines to guard against cuts:

- Keep any sharp objects, including knives, peelers, graters, food processor blades, scissors, nail clippers, and razors out of reach of children.
- Lock sharp objects away if there is a confused client in the home.
- If you are preparing food, cut away from yourself, use a cutting board, and keep your fingers out of the way.
- Know proper first aid for cuts.

Choking. Choking can occur when eating, drinking or swallowing medication. Babies and young children who put objects in their mouths are at great risk of choking. People who are weak, ill, or unconscious may choke on their own saliva. A person's tongue can also become swollen and obstruct the airway. Follow these guidelines to guard against choking:

- Keep small objects out of reach of babies and small children.

- Cut food into bite-sized pieces for clients who have trouble with utensils and for children.

- Position infants on their backs for sleeping after feeding. Infants should sleep on their backs to prevent sudden infant death syndrome (SIDS). Never put pillows, small toys, or other objects in a crib.

- Clients should eat in as upright a position as possible to avoid choking. Elderly clients with swallowing difficulties may have a special diet with liquids thickened to the consistency of honey. Thickened liquids are easier to swallow. See Section VI for more information on swallowing problems and thickened liquids.

Fire. Follow these guidelines to guard against fire:

- Roll up clients' sleeves and avoid loose clothing when client may be cooking or around the stove.

- Store potholders, dish towels, and other flammable kitchen items away from the stove.

- Never store cookies, candy, or other items that may attract children above or near the stove.

- Discourage careless smoking and smoking in bed. If clients must smoke, check to be sure that cigarettes are extinguished. Empty ashtrays frequently. Before emptying ashtrays, make sure there are no hot ashes or hot matches in ashtray.

- Stay in or near the kitchen when anything is cooking or baking.

- Do not leave the dryer on when you leave the house. Lint can catch fire.

- Turn off space heaters when no one is home or everyone is asleep.

- Be sure there are working smoke alarms.

- Have fire extinguishers on hand. Every home should have a fire extinguisher in the kitchen. Know where fire extinguisher is stored and how to operate it:

- **P**ull the pin.

- **A**im at the base of the fire when spraying.

- **S**queeze the handle.

- **S**weep back and forth at the base of the fire.

In case of fire, RACE is a good rule to follow:

- **R**emove clients from danger.
- **A**ctivate 911.
- **C**ontain fire if possible.
- **E**xtinguish, or call fire department to extinguish.

In addition, follow these guidelines for helping clients and family members exit the home safely:

- Remain calm.
- Be sure all family members know how to exit in case of fire, and have a designated meeting place outside the home.
- If windows or doors have locking bars, keep keys in the lock or close by to allow escape in case of fire. Mark windows of children's rooms with stickers that indicate a child sleeps in the room.
- Remove anything blocking a window or door that could be used as a fire exit.
- If clothing catches fire, do not run. Drop to the ground and roll to extinguish flames.
- Do not try to put out a large fire. Get out of the house and call for emergency help.

Travel Safety

Auto accidents. Since you may be driving to and from clients' homes, you will need to protect your safety. Follow these guidelines:

- **Plan your route.** Trying to read a map or directions while driving can be very dangerous. When you must drive to a new location, study the map or directions before you start your car.
- **Minimize distractions.** Paying attention to the road can help you avoid accidents. Keep your eyes on the road and your hands on the wheel. If music is distracting, do not listen in the car. Do not talk on your cell phone.
- **Use turn signals.** Using your turn signals lets other drivers know what you are planning to do. Always use turn signals when preparing to turn or change lanes.
- **Use caution when backing up.** Many accidents occur when drivers back up. When you back up, look around you carefully. Turn your head to both sides and look behind your car.

- **Drive at a safe speed.** Follow speed limits to be sure you are not driving too fast. Road conditions such as ice or heavy rain may mean you have to drive at a slower speed.

- **Always wear your seat belt.** Although it may not help you avoid an accident, it will certainly help protect you if an accident occurs.

- **Keep your driver's license, valid car insurance, and proof of registration with you** in case you're ever in an accident or stopped by police.

If an assignment takes you to an area where crime is a problem, use caution. If you are using public transportation, be alert at all times. Follow these guidelines to help avoid trouble:

- Park in well-lit areas, as close as possible to the home you are visiting.

- Try to leave valuables at home when you must work in a dangerous area.

- If possible, do not take your purse with you. If you must take it, hold your purse or bag tightly, close to your body.

- Lock your car and do not leave any valuables in it.

- Walk confidently. Look as though you know where you are going.

- Carry a whistle so you can make a loud noise to startle an attacker and get help.

- Carry your keys in your hand to unlock your car as soon as you arrive.

- Do not sit in your car, even with the doors locked. Drive away as soon as you reach your car.

- Try to avoid unsafe areas after dark.

- If you are concerned about your safety in a particular area, leave the area immediately. Contact your supervisor.

- Do not approach a home where strangers are hanging around. Go to the nearest phone in a safe area. Call your supervisor.

- Call your client before you visit so they know approximately when to expect you.

- Never enter a vacant home.

- If necessary, ask your supervisor to arrange for an escort or another care provider to go with you.

- Be sure someone knows your schedule. Call the office at the end of your work day.

7. Emergencies

Medical Emergencies

Medical emergencies may be caused by accidents or sudden illnesses. In this section you will learn how to respond to medical emergencies. Heart attacks, stroke, diabetic emergencies, choking, automobile accidents, and gunshot wounds are all medical emergencies. Severe falls, burns, and cuts can also be emergencies.

In an emergency, try to remain calm, act quickly, and communicate clearly. Knowing these steps will help:

Assess the situation. Try to find out what has happened. Make sure you are not in danger. Notice the time.

Assess the victim. Ask the injured or ill person what has happened. If the person cannot respond, he may be unconscious. Determine whether the person is conscious. Tap the person and ask if he is all right. Speak loudly. Use the person's name if you know it. If there is no response, assume the person is unconscious. Call for help right away, or send someone else to call.

If a person is conscious and able to speak, then he is breathing and has a pulse. Talk with the person about what happened. Check the person for injury. Look for severe bleeding, changes in consciousness, irregular breathing, unusual color or feel to the skin, swollen places on the body, medical alert tags, and anything the client says is painful. If any of these exist, you may need medical help. Always get help before doing anything else.

If the injured or ill person is conscious, he may be frightened. Listen to the person. Tell him what is being done to help him. Be calm and confident. Tell him that he is being taken care of.

When in doubt about calling for help, call! If you need to call emergency medical services, call 911 or dial 0 for the operator to get emergency medical services. If you are alone, make the call yourself. If you are not alone, shout for help and have someone make the call for you and then return to you.

When calling emergency services, be prepared to give the following information:

- the phone number and address of emergency, including exact directions or landmarks if necessary
- the person's condition, including any medical background you know
- your name and position
- details of any first aid being given

If the person is breathing, has a normal pulse, is normally responsive, and is not bleeding severely, you may not need to call for emergency services. If a client has fallen, been burned, or cut himself but the damage seems to be minor, call your supervisor. Let the person answering the phone know that you are with a client and an accident has occurred. If your supervisor is not available, another member of the care team may be able to help you.

Once the emergency is over, you will need to document it in your notes. Complete an incident report. Try to remember as many details as you can. Report the facts only. Knowing what information you will have to document will help you remember the important facts. Documenting emergencies accurately is very important to you and your agency.

Cardiopulmonary resuscitation (CPR) is the medical procedures used when a person's heart or lungs have stopped working. CPR is used until medical help arrives. Quick action is necessary. CPR must be started immediately. Only properly trained people should perform CPR. Your agency will probably arrange for you to be trained in CPR. If not, ask about American Heart Association or Red Cross CPR training, or contact one of these agencies yourself. CPR is an important skill to learn. If you are not trained, do not attempt to perform CPR. Performing CPR incorrectly can further injure a person.

This book is **not** a CPR course. The following is a brief review for people who have had CPR training.

1 Check to see if the person is responsive. Gently shake the person and shout, "Are you okay?"

2 If there is no response, call 911 immediately or send someone to call 911. Stay calm.

3 Kneel at the person's side near his or her head to start CPR.

4 Open the airway. Tilt the head back slightly. Lift the chin with one hand while pushing down on the forehead with the other hand (head tilt-chin lift method).

5 Hold the airway open and check for breathing:

- Look for the chest to rise and fall.

- Listen for sounds of breathing. Put your ear near the person's nose and mouth.

- Feel for the person's breath on your cheek.

6 If the person is not breathing, you will have to breathe for the person. Give two rescue breaths. To give rescue breaths:

- Pinch the nose to keep air from escaping. Cover the person's mouth completely with your mouth.

- If a barrier device, such as a special face mask, is available, use it to give rescue breathing.

- Blow into the person's mouth slowly. Watch for the chest to rise. Blow two full breaths, about two seconds each. Turn your head to the side to listen for air. If the chest does not rise when you give a rescue breath, reopen the airway. Use the head tilt-chin lift method. Try to give rescue breaths again.

7 After giving rescue breaths, look for signs of response. The person may start moving, breathing normally, or coughing. If you do not see a response, give 15 chest compressions. Do this only if you have been trained to do so. Be sure the person is lying flat on a hard surface. To give chest compressions:

- Find the lower end of the person's sternum. Do this by following the rib cage up to the center of the chest.

- Place your index finger next to your middle finger where the ribs meet the sternum. Place the heel of your other hand next to the upper finger over the lower half of the sternum.

- Place the heel of your other hand on top of the positioned hand. Extend or interlace your fingers. Make sure your fingers are kept off the chest. Position your body directly over your hands. Keep your elbows straight. Look down at your hands.

- Use the heel of your hands to give 15 chest compressions. Push in 1 1/2 to 2 inches with each compression. Allow the chest to relax between compressions. Do not take your hands off the chest between compressions.

8 Give two more rescue breaths followed by 15 compressions. After about a minute of CPR, check for signs of response. If you see signs of response, stop compressions. Continue to provide rescue breathing as necessary (one breath every five seconds).

When medical help arrives follow their directions. Assist them as necessary. Report details of the incident.

Choking

When something is blocking the tube through which air enters the lungs, the person has an obstructed airway. When people are choking, they usually put their hands to their throat and cough. As long as a person can speak, cough, or breathe, do nothing. Encourage him to cough as forcefully as possible to get the object out. Stay with the person at all times, until he stops choking or can no longer speak, breathe, or cough. Do not hit him on the back. If a person can no longer speak, cough, or breathe, or turns blue, call 911 immediately. After calling 911 return to the person. Time is of extreme importance. The Heimlich maneuver is a procedure used for choking. It uses abdominal thrusts to move the blockage upward, out of the throat.

Heimlich maneuver for the conscious person

1. Stand behind the person. Bring your arms under his arms. Wrap your arms around the person's waist.

2. Make a fist with one hand. Place the flat, thumb side of the fist against the person's abdomen, above the navel but below the breastbone.

3. Grasp the fist with your other hand. Pull both hands toward you and up, quickly and forcefully.

4. Repeat until the object is pushed out or the person loses consciousness.

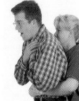

Insulin Shock and Diabetic Coma

Insulin shock and diabetic coma are complications of diabetes that can be life-threatening. Insulin shock, or hypoglycemia (hye-poh-glye-SEE-mee-a), can result from either too much insulin or too little food. It occurs when insulin is given and the person skips a meal or does not eat all the food required. Even when a regular amount of food is eaten, physical activity may rapidly absorb the food. This causes too much insulin to be in the body. Vomiting and diarrhea may also lead to insulin shock in people with diabetes.

The first signs of insulin shock include feeling weak or different, nervousness, dizziness, and perspiration (see list below for further signs). These signal that the client needs food in a form that can be rapidly absorbed. A lump of sugar, a hard candy, or a glass of orange juice should be consumed right away. A diabetic should always have a quick source of sugar handy. Contact your supervisor if the client has shown early signs of insulin shock.

The following are signs and symptoms of insulin shock:

- hunger
- weakness
- rapid pulse
- headache
- low blood pressure
- perspiration
- cold, clammy skin
- confusion
- trembling
- nervousness
- blurred vision
- numbness of the lips and tongue
- unconsciousness

Having too little insulin causes diabetic coma, also known as acidosis (a-sid-OH-sis) or hyperglycemia (high-per-glye-SEE-mee-a). It can result from undiagnosed diabetes, not enough insulin, eating too much, not getting enough exercise, and physical or emotional stress.

The signs of diabetic coma include increased thirst or urination, abdominal pain, deep or difficult breathing, and breath that smells sweet or fruity (see complete list of symptoms below). Call your supervisor immediately if you suspect your client is experiencing diabetic coma or insulin shock. Know and follow your agency's policies and procedures for when to call emergency services.

Other signs and symptoms of diabetic coma include the following:

- hunger
- weakness
- rapid, weak pulse
- headache
- low blood pressure

- dry skin
- flushed cheeks
- drowsiness
- slow, deep, and labored breathing
- nausea and vomiting
- abdominal pain
- sweet, fruity breath odor
- air hunger, or client gasping for air and being unable to catch his breath
- unconsciousness

Refer to the Special Conditions section for more information on diabetes.

CVA or Stroke

A cerebrovascular accident (CVA), or stroke, is caused when blood supply to the brain is suddenly cut off by a clot or a ruptured blood vessel. A stroke may be preceded by symptoms. These symptoms include dizziness, ringing in the ears, headache, nausea, vomiting, slurring of words, and loss of memory. These symptoms should be reported immediately.

A transient ischemic attack (TRAN-see-ent is-KEE-mik a-TAK), or TIA, is a warning sign of a CVA. It is the result of a temporary lack of oxygen in the brain. Symptoms may last up to 24 hours. Symptoms include tingling, weakness, or some loss of movement in an arm or leg. These symptoms should not be ignored. Report any of these to your supervisor immediately.

Signs that a stroke is occurring include any of the following:

- loss of consciousness
- redness in the face
- noisy breathing
- seizures
- loss of bowel and bladder control
- hemiplegia (hem-i-PLEE-jee-a)
- hemiparesis (hem-i-pa-REE-sis)
- aphasia (a-FAY-see-a)
- use of inappropriate words

- elevated blood pressure

- slow pulse rate

Refer to the Special Conditions section for more information on strokes.

Myocardial Infarction or Heart Attack

When blood flow to the heart is completely blocked, oxygen and nutrients fail to reach the cells in that region. Waste products are not removed and the muscle cell dies. This is called a myocardial infarction (mye-oh-KAR-dee-al in-FARK-shun) or MI, or heart attack. The area of dead tissue may be large or small, depending on the artery involved.

A myocardial infarction is an emergency that can result in serious heart damage or death. The following are signs and symptoms of MI:

- sudden, severe pain in the chest, usually on the left side or in the center behind the sternum

- a feeling of indigestion or heartburn

- nausea and vomiting

- dyspnea (DISP-nee-a) or difficulty breathing

- dizziness

- pale, gray, or cyanotic (sye-a-NOT-ik) skin; cyanotic skin is a bluish color, indicating lack of oxygen

- perspiration

- cold and clammy skin

- weak and irregular pulse rate

- low blood pressure

- anxiety and a sense of impending doom

- denial of a heart problem

The pain of a heart attack is commonly described as a crushing, pressing, squeezing, stabbing, piercing pain, or "like someone is sitting on my chest." The pain may radiate down the inside of the left arm. A person may also feel it in the neck and/or in the jaw. The pain usually does not go away.

You must take immediate action if a client has any of these symptoms. Follow these steps:

1 Call or have someone call emergency services. Call your supervisor.

2 Place the client in a comfortable position. Encourage him to rest, and reassure him that you will not leave him alone.

3 Loosen clothing around the neck.

4 Do not give the client liquids or food.

5 If the client takes heart medication, such as nitroglycerin, find the medication and offer it to him. Never place medication in someone's mouth.

6 Monitor the client's breathing and pulse. If the client stops breathing or has no pulse, perform rescue breathing or CPR only if you are trained to do so.

7 Stay with the client until help arrives.

8 Report and document the incident properly.

Refer to the Special Conditions section for more information on MIs or heart attacks.

Disaster Guidelines

Home health aides need to be knowledgeable and responsible during a disaster. An emergency or disaster may occur during working hours. You will be expected to know how to respond in a calm and intelligent manner. Disasters can include fire, flood, earthquake, hurricane, tornado, or severe weather. The following guidelines apply in any disaster situation:

- Remain calm.

- Listen to radio or television bulletins to keep informed. A battery-powered radio will allow you to stay informed if the power goes out.

- If a disaster is forecast (for example, a tornado or hurricane), be ready. Wear appropriate clothing and shoes. Have family members dressed and ready in case evacuation is necessary.

- Stay in contact with your supervisor or others if possible. Let someone know where you are, what conditions are, and where you will go if you must evacuate.

- Locate disaster supplies. Ideally, a disaster supplies kit should be assembled before disaster strikes. See below.

Emergency Supplies

Keep enough supplies in your home to meet your needs for at least three days. Assemble a disaster supply kit with items you may need in an evacuation. Store these supplies in sturdy, easy-to-carry containers such as backpacks, duffel bags or covered trash containers.

INCLUDE:

- A three-day supply of water (one gallon per person per day) and food that will not spoil
- One change of clothing and footwear per person, and one blanket or sleeping bag per person
- A first aid kit that includes your family's prescription medications
- Emergency tools, including a battery-powered radio, flashlight, and plenty of extra batteries
- An extra set of car keys and a credit card, cash, or traveler's checks
- Sanitation supplies
- Special items for infant, elderly, or disabled family members
- An extra pair of glasses
- Important family documents in a waterproof container

The disasters you may experience will depend on where you live. Know the proper action to take to protect yourself and your client. During natural disasters, most agencies rely on local or state management groups to assume overall responsibility for the ill and disabled. Each agency has a local and area-specific disaster plan. Know your agency's plan.

You will be required to apply general guidelines as well as specific guidelines for the area in which you work. For example, a HHA working where hurricanes occur, such as Florida, needs to know the guidelines for hurricanes preparedness, as well as for storms and fires. The following guidelines are separated by the type of disaster. They can be used in any particular geographical area that applies to your specific job and location. Always keep the radio or television on to get the latest information.

Tornadoes

In the case of tornadoes, follow these guidelines:

- Seek shelter inside, such as steel-framed or concrete buildings.

- Stay away from windows.
- Stand in the hallway or in a basement, or take cover under heavy furniture.
- Do not stay in a mobile home or trailer.
- Lie as flat as possible.

Lightning

If outdoors, follow these guidelines:

- Avoid the largest objects such as trees and open spaces.
- Stay out of the water.
- Seek shelter in buildings.
- Stay away from metal fences, doors or other objects.
- Avoid holding metal objects, such as golf clubs, in your hands.
- Stay in automobiles.
- CPR is safe to perform because lightning victims carry no electricity.

If indoors, stay inside and away from open doors and windows. Avoid using electrical equipment such as hair dryers and televisions. Do not use the phone.

Floods

In the case of floods, follow these guidelines:

- Fill the bathtub with fresh water.
- Board up windows.
- Evacuate if advised to do so.
- Check the fuel level in automobiles.
- Have a portable battery-operated radio, flashlight, and cooking equipment available.
- Do not drink water or eat food that has been contaminated with flood water.
- Do not handle electrical equipment.
- Do not turn off gas yourself, but ask the gas company to do so.

Blackouts

In the case of blackouts, follow these guidelines:

- In a facility you will have access to either a generator or a flashlight.

- In a home, ask your client where the emergency supplies are kept. Take prompt action to keep calm and provide light.

- Use a back-up pack for electrical medical equipment such as an IV pump. Back-up packs do not last more than 24 hours, so call emergency services.

Hurricanes

In the case of hurricanes, follow these guidelines:

- Know what category the hurricane is and track the expected path.

- Know which clients must go to shelters, nursing homes, or hospitals, and which need assistance.

- Call your employer for instructions.

- Contact your clients if instructed to do so.

- Fill the bathtub with fresh water.

- Board up windows.

- Evacuate if advised to do so.

- Check the fuel level in automobiles.

- Have a portable battery-operated radio, flashlight, and cooking equipment available.

- Be aware of people with special needs.

- High-risk people include the elderly and those unable to evacuate on their own. High-risk areas include mobile homes or trailers.

III
Understanding Your Clients

8. Culture and Family

Basic Human Needs

People have different genes, physical appearances, cultural backgrounds, ages, and social or financial positions. But all human beings have the same basic physical needs:

- food and water

- protection and shelter

- activity

- sleep and rest

- safety

- comfort, especially freedom from pain

We also have psychosocial needs, which involve social interaction, emotions, intellect, and spirituality. Psychosocial needs are not as easy to define as physical needs. However, all human beings have the following psychosocial needs:

- love and affection

- acceptance by others

- security

- self-reliance and independence in daily living

- interaction with other people

- accomplishments and self-esteem

Health and well-being affect how well psychosocial needs are met. Stress and frustration occur when basic needs are not met. This can lead to fear, anxiety, anger, aggression, withdrawal, indifference, and depression. Stress can also cause physical problems that may eventually lead to illness.

Abraham Maslow, a researcher of human behavior, wrote about human physical and psychosocial needs. He arranged these needs into an order of importance. He thought that physical needs must be met before psychosocial needs can be met. His theory is called "Maslow's Hierarchy of Needs."

Cultural Differences

People come from many different cultural backgrounds and religious traditions. You will take care of clients with different backgrounds and traditions than your own. It is important to respect and value each person as an individual. Sometimes it is easier to accept different practices or beliefs if you understand a little about them.

There are so many different cultures that they cannot all be listed here. A culture is a system of behaviors people learn from the group of people they grow up and live with. One might talk about American culture being different from Japanese culture. But within American culture there are thousands of different groups with their own cultures: Japanese-Americans, African-Americans, and Native Americans, just to name a few. Even people from a particular region, state, or city can be said to have a different culture. The culture of the South is not the same as the culture of New York City.

Cultural background affects how friendly people are to strangers. It can affect how they feel about having you in their houses, or how close they want you to stand to them when talking. Be sensitive to your clients' backgrounds. You cannot expect to be treated the same way by all your clients. Adjust your behavior around some of your clients. Regardless of their background, you must treat all clients with respect and professionalism. Expect them to treat you respectfully as well.

Religious differences also influence the way people behave. Religion can be very important in people's lives, particularly when they are ill or dying. You must respect the religious beliefs and practices of your clients, even if they are different from your own. Never question your clients' religious beliefs. Do not discuss your own beliefs with them.

Be aware of specific practices that might affect your work. Many religious beliefs include dietary restrictions. These are rules about what and when followers can eat and drink. Check with your agency if you are unsure about planning and preparing meals for clients. Be aware of any dietary restrictions. Honor them.

Some people's backgrounds may make them less comfortable being touched by others. Be sensitive to your clients' feelings. You must touch clients in order to do your job. However, recognize that some clients feel more comfortable when there is little physical contact.

Families

Families are the most important unit within our social system. Families play a huge role in most people's lives. Some examples of family types are listed below.

- Single-parent families include one parent with a child or children.

- Nuclear families include two parents with a child or children.

- Blended families include widowed or divorced parents who have remarried, with children from previous marriages as well as from this marriage.

- Multigenerational families include parents, children, and grandparents.

- Extended families may include aunts, uncles, cousins, or even friends.

- Families may also be made up of unmarried couples of the same sex or opposite sexes, with or without children.

Family members help in many ways:

- helping clients make care decisions

- communicating with the care team

- providing daily care when home health aide is not present

- giving support and encouragement

- connecting the client to the outside world

- giving assurance to dying clients that family memories and traditions will be valued and carried on

9. Body Systems

Each system in the body has a condition under which it works best. Homeostasis (hoh-mee-oh-STAY-sis) is the name for the condition in which all of the body's systems are working their best. To be in homeostasis, the body's metabolism, or physical and chemical processes, must be operating at a steady level. When disease or injury occur, the body's metabolism is disturbed. Homeostasis is lost. Changes in metabolic (me-tah-BOL-ic) processes are called signs and symptoms. Each system in the body has its own unique structure and function. The body's systems can be broken down in different ways. In this book we divide the human body into ten body systems:

1 Integumentary (in-teg-you-MEN-tar-ee), or skin

2 Musculoskeletal (mus-kyoo-lo-SKEL-e-tal)

3 Nervous

4 Circulatory (SER-kyoo-la-tor-ee) or cardiovascular (kar-dee-oh-VAS-kyoo-lar)

5 Respiratory (RES-spir-a-tor-ee)

6 Urinary (YOOR-i-nayr-ee)

7 Gastrointestinal or digestive

8 Endocrine (EN-doh-krin)

9 Reproductive

10 Immune and Lymphatic (lim-FAT-ik)

Body systems are made up of organs. Organs are made up of tissues. Tissues are made up of groups of cells that perform a similar function. For example, in the circulatory system, the heart is one of the organs. It is made up of tissues and cells. Cells are the building blocks of bodies. Living cells divide, develop, and die, renewing the tissues and organs of the body systems.

Common Disorders/Observing and Reporting

1 The Integumentary System

The largest organ and system in the body is the skin, a natural protective covering, or integument. Skin prevents injury to internal organs. It also protects the body against entry of bacteria or germs. Skin also prevents the loss of too much water, which is essential to life. Skin is made up of tissues and glands (structures that secrete fluids).

The skin is also a sense organ that feels heat, cold, pain, touch, and pressure. It then tells the brain what it is feeling. Body temperature is regulated in the skin, which has blood vessels that dilate when the outside temperature is too high. This brings more blood to the body surface to cool it off. The same blood vessels constrict when the outside temperature is too cold. By restricting the amount of blood reaching the skin, the blood vessels help the body retain heat.

INTEGUMENTARY SYSTEM: COMMON DISORDERS

• Pressure sores, or decubitus (dee-KYOO-bi-tus) ulcers

INTEGUMENTARY SYSTEM: OBSERVING AND REPORTING

Observe and report the following signs and symptoms immediately:

- rashes or scales

- bruising

- cuts, boils, sores, wounds, abrasions

- changes in color or moistness/dryness

- swelling

- scalp or hair changes

- skin that appears different from normal or that has changed

2 The Musculoskeletal System

Muscles, bones, ligaments, tendons, and cartilage give the body shape and structure. They work together to allow the body to move. Exercise is important for improving and maintaining both physical and mental health. Range of motion (ROM) exercises can help prevent loss of self-esteem, depression, pneumonia, urinary tract infection, constipation, blood clots, dulling of the senses, and muscle atrophy or contractures.

MUSCULOSKELETAL SYSTEM: COMMON DISORDERS

- Fractures

- Osteoporosis (os-tee-oh-poh-ROH-sis)

- Arthritis

MUSCULOSKELETAL SYSTEM: OBSERVING AND REPORTING

Observe and report the following signs and symptoms immediately:

- changes in ability to perform routine movements and activities

- any changes in clients' ability to perform ROM exercises

- pain during movement

- any new or increased swelling of joints

- white, shiny, red, or warm areas over a joint

- bruising

- aches and pains clients report to you

3 The Nervous System

The nervous system is the control center and message center of the body. It controls and coordinates all body functions. The nervous system also senses and interprets information from the environment outside the human body.

CENTRAL NERVOUS SYSTEM: COMMON DISORDERS

- Dementia, including Alzheimer's disease
- Cerebrovascular (se-ree-broh-VAS-kyoo-lar) accident (CVA), or stroke
- Parkinson's disease
- Multiple sclerosis (skle-ROH-sis)
- Epilepsy
- Cerebral palsy (SER-eh-bral PAL-zee)
- Head and spinal cord injuries

CENTRAL NERVOUS SYSTEM: OBSERVING AND REPORTING

Observe and report the following signs and symptoms immediately:

- fatigue or pain with movement or exercise
- shaking or trembling
- inability to speak clearly
- inability to move one side of body
- disturbance or change in vision or hearing
- changes in eating patterns or fluid intake
- difficulty swallowing
- bowel and bladder changes
- depression or mood changes
- memory loss or confusion
- violent behavior
- any unusual or unexplained change in behavior
- decreased ability to perform ADLs

The Nervous System: Sense Organs

The eyes, ears, nose, tongue, and skin are the body's major sense organs. They are considered part of the central nervous system because they contain receptors that receive impulses from the environment. They relay these impulses to nerves.

EYES AND EARS: COMMON DISORDERS

- Cataracts (KAT-a-rakts)

- Glaucoma (glaw-KOH-ma)
- Otitis media (oh-TYE-tis MEE-dee-a)
- Deafness
- Vertigo

EYES AND EARS: OBSERVING AND REPORTING

Observe and report the following signs and symptoms immediately:

- changes in vision or hearing
- signs of infection
- dizziness
- client complaints of pain in eyes or ears

4 The Circulatory or Cardiovascular System

The circulatory system is made up of the heart, blood vessels, and blood. The heart pumps blood through the blood vessels to the cells. The blood carries food, oxygen, and other substances that cells need to function properly.

The circulatory system performs the following major functions:

- supplying food, oxygen, and hormones to cells
- producing and supplying antibodies and other infection-fighting blood cells
- removing waste products from cells
- controlling body temperature

CIRCULATORY SYSTEM: COMMON DISORDERS

- Atherosclerosis (ath-er-oh-skle-ROH-sis)
- Myocardial infarction (MI), or heart attack
- Angina pectoris (an-JYE-na PEK-tor-is)
- Hypertension, or high blood pressure
- Congestive heart failure
- Peripheral vascular disease

CIRCULATORY SYSTEM: OBSERVING AND REPORTING

Observe and report the following signs and symptoms immediately:

- changes in pulse rate
- weakness, fatigue

- loss of ability to perform activities of daily living (ADLs)
- swelling of hands and feet
- pale or blue appearance of hands, feet, or lips
- chest pain
- weight gain
- shortness of breath, changes in breathing patterns, inability to catch breath
- severe headache
- inactivity (which can lead to circulatory problems)

5 The Respiratory System

Respiration, the body taking in oxygen and removing carbon dioxide, involves breathing in (inspiration), and breathing out (expiration). The lungs accomplish this process.

The respiratory system has two functions:

1 It brings oxygen into the body.
2 It eliminates carbon dioxide produced as the body uses oxygen.

RESPIRATORY SYSTEM: COMMON DISORDERS

- Asthma (AZ-ma)
- Upper respiratory infection (URI), or a cold
- Bronchitis (brong-KYE-tis)
- Pneumonia (new-MOH-nee-a)
- Emphysema (em-fi-SEE-ma)
- Lung cancer
- Tuberculosis (too-ber-kyoo-LOH-sis)
- Chronic obstructive pulmonary disease (COPD)

RESPIRATORY SYSTEM: OBSERVING AND REPORTING

Observe and report the following signs and symptoms immediately:

- change in respiratory rate
- shallow breathing or breathing through pursed lips
- coughing or wheezing
- nasal congestion or discharge
- sore throat, difficulty swallowing, or swollen tonsils

- the need to sit after mild exertion
- the need to rest on two pillows
- pale or bluish color of the lips and extremities
- pain in the chest area
- discolored sputum (green, yellow, blood-tinged, or gray)

6 The Urinary System

The urinary system has two vital functions:

1 Through urine, it eliminates waste products created by the cells.
2 It maintains the water balance in the body.

URINARY SYSTEM: COMMON DISORDERS

- Urinary tract infection (UTI), or cystitis (sis-TYE-tis)
- Calculi (KAL-kyoo-lye)
- Nephritis (ne-FRYE-tis)
- Renovascular hypertension (ree-noh-VAS- kyoo-lar high-per-TEN-shun)
- Chronic kidney failure, or uremia (you-REE-mee-a)
- Benign prostatic hypertrophy (be-NINE pros-TAT-ik HIGH-per-troh-fee)

URINARY SYSTEM: OBSERVING AND REPORTING

Observe and report the following signs and symptoms immediately:

- weight loss or gain
- swelling in the upper or lower extremities
- painful urination or burning during urination
- changes in the characteristics of urine, such as cloudiness, odor, or color
- changes in frequency and amount of urination
- swelling in the abdominal/bladder area
- client complaining that bladder feels full or painful
- incontinence/dribbling
- pain in the kidney or back/flank region
- inadequate fluid intake

7 The Gastrointestinal (GI) System

The gastrointestinal system has two functions: digestion and elimination. Digestion is the process of preparing food physically and chemically so that it can be absorbed into the cells. Elimination is the process of expelling solid wastes made up of food waste products that are not absorbed into the cells.

GASTROINTESTINAL SYSTEM: COMMON DISORDERS

- Heartburn
- Gastroesophageal reflux disease (GERD)
- Peptic ulcers
- Constipation
- Diarrhea
- Hepatitis
- Ulcerative colitis (UL-ser-a-tiv koh-LYE-tis)
- Colitis
- Colorectal (koh-loh-REK-tal) cancer
- Hemorrhoids

GASTROINTESTINAL SYSTEM: OBSERVING AND REPORTING

Observe and report the following signs and symptoms immediately:

- difficulty swallowing or chewing (including denture problems or mouth sores)
- fecal incontinence (losing control of bowels)
- weight gain/weight loss
- anorexia (loss of appetite)
- abdominal pain and cramping
- diarrhea
- nausea and vomiting (especially vomitus that looks like coffee grounds)
- constipation
- flatulence
- hiccups, belching
- abnormally-colored stool (bloody, black, or hard)
- heartburn
- poor nutritional intake

8 The Endocrine System

The endocrine system is made up of glands that secrete hormones. Hormones are chemicals that control many of the organs and body systems. They are carried in the blood to the various organs, where they perform the following functions:

- maintain homeostasis
- influence growth and development
- regulate levels of sugar in the blood
- regulate levels of calcium in the bones
- determine how fast cells burn food for energy

ENDOCRINE SYSTEM: COMMON DISORDERS

- Hyperthyroidism (high-per-THIGH-royd-ism)
- Hypothyroidism (high-poh-THIGH-royd-ism)
- Diabetes (dye-a-BEE-teez)

ENDOCRINE SYSTEM: OBSERVING AND REPORTING

Many endocrine illnesses can be treated with hormone supplements. These supplements must be given very precisely. For example, too much insulin administered to a diabetic can cause the sudden onset of insulin shock. Observe and report the following signs and symptoms:

- headache*
- weakness*
- blurred vision*
- dizziness*
- hunger*
- irritability*
- sweating*
- change in "normal" behavior*
- increased confusion*
- weight gain/weight loss
- loss of appetite/increased appetite
- increased thirst
- frequent urination

- dry skin
- sluggishness or fatigue
- hyperactivity

* indicates signs and symptoms that should be reported immediately

9 The Reproductive System

The reproductive system is made up of the reproductive organs, which are different in men and women. The reproductive system allows human beings to reproduce, or create new human life. Reproduction begins when a man's and woman's sex cells (sperm and ovum) join. These sex cells are formed in the male and female sex glands, called the gonads.

REPRODUCTIVE SYSTEM: COMMON DISORDERS

- Vaginitis (vaj-i-NYE-tis)
- Benign prostatic hypertrophy
- Chlamydia (kla-MID-ee- a)
- Syphilis (SIF-i-lis)
- Gonorrhea (gon-oh-REE-a)
- Herpes simplex II

REPRODUCTIVE SYSTEM: OBSERVING AND REPORTING

Observe and report the following signs and symptoms immediately:

- discomfort or difficulty with urination
- discharge from the penis or vagina
- swelling of the genitals
- changes in menstruation
- blood in urine or stool
- breast changes, including size, shape, lumps, or discharge from the nipple
- sores on the genitals
- client reports of impotence, or inability of male to have sexual intercourse
- client reports of painful intercourse

10 The Immune and Lymphatic Systems

The immune system protects the body from disease-causing bacteria, viruses, and organisms. The immune system protects the body in two ways. Nonspecific immunity protects the body from disease in general. Specific immunity protects against a particular disease that is invading the body at a given time.

The lymphatic system removes excess fluids and waste products from the body's tissues. It also helps the immune system fight infection.

IMMUNE AND LYMPHATIC SYSTEMS: COMMON DISORDERS

- HIV/AIDS
- Lymphoma (lim-FOH-ma)

IMMUNE AND LYMPHATIC SYSTEMS: OBSERVING AND REPORTING

Observe and report the following signs and symptoms immediately:

- recurring infections (such as pneumonia, diarrhea, and fevers)
- swelling of the lymph nodes
- increased fatigue

10. Human Development

Stages/Common Disorders

Everyone will go through the same stages of development during their lives. However, no two people will follow the exact same pattern or rate of development. Each client must be treated as an individual and a whole person who is growing and developing rather than someone who is merely ill or disabled.

Infancy, Birth to Twelve Months

Infants grow and develop very quickly. In one year a baby moves from total dependence on the caregiver to the relative independence of moving around, communicating basic needs, and feeding himself.

Physical development in infancy moves from the head down. For example, infants gain control over the muscles of the neck before they are able to control the muscles in their shoulders. Control over muscles in the trunk area, such as the shoulders, develops before control of the arms and legs. This head-to-toe sequence should be respected when caring for infants. For example, newborns must be supported at the shoulders, head, and neck, and babies who cannot sit or crawl should not be encouraged to stand or walk.

INFANCY: COMMON DISORDERS

- Prematurity
- Low birth weight
- Birth defects: Cerebral palsy, cystic fibrosis, Down syndrome
- Viral or bacterial infections
- Sudden infant death syndrome (SIDS)

Childhood

The Toddler Period, Ages One to Three

During the toddler years, children gain independence. One part of this independence is new control over their bodies. Toddlers learn to speak, gain coordination of their limbs, and gain control over their bladders and bowels.

Toddlers assert their new independence by exploring further and further from the caregiver. Poisons and other hazards, such as sharp objects, must be locked away.

Psychologically, toddlers learn that they are individuals, separate from their parents. Children at this age may try to control their parents. They may try to get what they want by throwing tantrums, whining, or refusing to cooperate. This is a key time for parents to establish rules and standards.

The Preschool Years, Ages Three to Six

Children in their preschool years develop skills that will help them become more independent and have social relationships. They develop vocabulary and language skills. They learn to play cooperatively in groups. They become more physically coordinated, and learn to care for themselves. Preschoolers also develop ways of relating to family members. They begin to learn right from wrong.

School-Age Children, Ages Six to Twelve

From ages six to about eight years, children's development is centered on cognitive (KOG-ni-tiv) (thinking and learning skills) and social development. As children enter school, they also explore the environment around them. They relate to other children through games, peer groups, and classroom activities. In these years, children learn to get along with each other. They also begin to behave in ways common to those of their sex. They begin to develop a conscience, morals, and self-esteem.

CHILDHOOD: COMMON DISORDERS

- Chicken pox
- Infections caused by viruses or bacteria
- Leukemia (loo-KEE-mee-a)
- Child abuse
- Measles, mumps, rubella, diphtheria, smallpox, whooping cough, polio (Most children are immunized against these disorders.)

Adolescence

Puberty

Puberty is the stage of growth when secondary sex characteristics appear. Also, reproductive organs begin to function due to the secretion of the reproductive hormones. The onset of puberty occurs between the ages of ten and sixteen for girls and twelve and fourteen for boys.

Adolescence, Ages Twelve to Eighteen

Many teenagers have a hard time adapting to the rapid changes that occur in their bodies after puberty. Peer acceptance is important to them. Because they see images of perfection in the media, adolescents may be afraid that they are unattractive or abnormal.

This concern for body image and peer acceptance, combined with changing hormones that influence moods, can cause adolescents to swing from one mood to another. Conflicting pressures develop as they remain dependent on their parents and yet need to express themselves socially and sexually. This can cause conflict and stress. Social interaction between members of the opposite sex becomes very important.

ADOLESCENCE: COMMON DISORDERS

- Eating disorders: anorexia, bulimia
- Sexually transmitted diseases (STDs)
- Teenage pregnancy
- Depression
- Trauma or accidental injury

Adulthood

Young Adulthood, Ages Eighteen to Forty

By the age of eighteen, most young adults have stopped growing.

Adopting a healthy lifestyle in these years can make life better now and prevent health problems in later adulthood. Psychological and social development continues, however. The developmental tasks of these years include choosing an appropriate education and an occupation or career, selecting a mate, learning to live with a mate or others, raising children, and developing a satisfying sex life.

Middle Adulthood: Forty to Sixty-five Years

In general, people in middle adulthood are more comfortable and stable than they were in previous stages. Many of their major life decisions have already been made. In the early years of middle adulthood people sometimes experience a "mid-life crisis." This is a period of unrest centered around an unconscious desire for change and for fulfillment of unmet goals.

Late Adulthood: Sixty-five Years and Older

Persons in late adulthood must adjust to the effects of aging. These effects or changes can include the loss of physical strength and health, death of loved ones, retirement, and preparation for their own death. Although the developmental tasks of this age appear to deal entirely with loss, solutions may involve new relationships, friendships, and interests.

The disorders you are most likely to see in this age group are discussed in Section V.

Aging

As a person ages, certain changes are considered normal changes of aging, including the following:

- skin is thinner, drier and more fragile
- muscles are not as strong
- bones become more brittle
- ability to think quickly and logically is affected
- senses of vision, hearing, taste and smell change
- heart is less efficient
- more frequent urinary elimination
- less efficient digestion
- changes in the production of hormones
- weakened immunity

- mild forgetfulness
- lifestyle changes

There are also changes which are NOT considered normal changes of aging and should be reported to your supervisor. These include:

- disorientation
- difficulty concentrating
- depression
- dementia, or a loss of mental abilities that interferes with ADLs
- confusion
- suicidal thoughts
- insomnia

Keep in mind that this is not a complete list. **Your job is to report any change, normal or not.**

Death

Death can occur suddenly and without warning, or it can be expected. Older people, or people with terminal illnesses, may have time to prepare for death. A terminal illness is a disease or condition that will eventually cause death. Preparing for death is a process that involves the dying person's emotions and behavior.

Dr. Elisabeth Kubler-Ross researched and wrote about the process of dying. Her book, *On Death and Dying*, describes five stages that dying people and their families or friends may experience before death. These five stages are described below.

- **Denial.** People in the denial stage may refuse to believe they are dying. They often believe a mistake has been made.
- **Anger.** Once they start to face the possibility of their death, people become angry that they are dying.
- **Bargaining.** Once people have begun to believe that they really are dying, they may make promises to God or somehow try to bargain for their recovery.
- **Depression.** As dying people become physically weaker and symptoms of the illness get worse, they may become deeply sad or depressed.
- **Acceptance.** Some people who are dying are eventually able to accept

death and prepare for it. They may make plans for their last days or for the ceremonies that may follow.

As with dying, grieving is an individual process. No two people will grieve in exactly the same way. Clergy, counselors, or social workers can provide help for people who are grieving. Family members or friends may have any of the following reactions to the death of a loved one:

- shock
- denial
- anger
- guilt
- regret
- sadness
- loneliness

Death is a very sensitive topic. Many people find it hard to discuss death. Feelings and attitudes about death can be influenced by many factors, such as:

- experience with death
- personality type
- religious beliefs
- cultural background

Common signs of approaching death include the following:

- blurred and failing vision
- unfocused eyes
- impaired speech
- diminished sense of touch
- loss of movement, muscle tone, and feeling
- rising or below-normal body temperature
- decreasing blood pressure
- weak pulse that is abnormally slow or rapid
- slow, irregular respirations or rapid, shallow respirations
- cold, pale skin
- mottling, spotting, or blotching of skin caused by poor circulation
- perspiration
- incontinence
- disorientation or confusion

GUIDELINES: CARING FOR THE DYING CLIENT

- **Diminished senses.** Keep room softly lighted without glare. Hearing is usually the last sense to go, so speak in a normal tone. Tell client about any procedures that are being done or what is happening in the room. Observe body language to anticipate client's needs.

- **Care of the mouth.** Give mouth care frequently. If client is unconscious, give mouth care every two hours. Apply lubricant, such as lip balm, to the lips.

- **Skin care.** Give bed baths and incontinence care as needed. Bathe perspiring clients often. Sheets and clothes should be changed for comfort. Skin care to prevent pressure sores is important.

- **Comfort.** Observe for signs of pain. Frequent changes of position, back massage, skin care, mouth care and proper body alignment may help.

- **Environment.** Display favorite objects and photographs for client. Make sure room is appropriately lighted and well ventilated.

- **Emotional and spiritual support.** Listen to client if she wishes to talk. Touch is important. Some clients may seek spiritual comfort from clergy members.

GUIDELINES: POSTMORTEM CARE

- Bathe the body. Be gentle to avoid bruising. Place drainage pads where needed. Follow Standard Precautions.

- Check with family about how to dress client and whether to remove jewelry.

- Do not remove any tubes or other equipment.

- Put dentures back in the mouth and close the mouth.

- Close the eyes carefully.

- Position the body on the back with legs straight, arms folded across the abdomen. Place a small pillow under the head.

- Strip the bed after body has been removed.

- Open windows to air room, as appropriate, and straighten up.

- Arrange personal items carefully so they are not lost.

- Document according to your agency's policy.

Respect the wishes of family and friends. Be sensitive to their needs after death occurs. Only perform assigned tasks.

Hospice Care

Hospice care is the term used for the special care that a dying person needs. Hospice care may be provided in a hospital, a special care facility, or in the home. A hospice can be any location where a person who is dying is treated with dignity by caregivers who provide for their physical, emotional, social, and spiritual needs. Besides pain relief, comfort, personal care, and emotional and spiritual support, clients who are dying also need to feel some independence for as long as possible. Caregivers should allow clients to retain as much control over their lives as possible. Eventually, caregivers may have to meet all of the client's basic needs.

Other attitudes and skills useful when providing hospice care include the following:

- Be a good listener. Do not push someone to talk, though.
- Respect privacy and independence.
- Be sensitive to individual needs. Ask how you can be of help.
- Be aware of your own feelings.
- Follow the plan of care.

In home care, goals will focus on the client's recovery, or on the client's ability to care for him- or herself as much as possible. In hospice care, however, the goals of care are the comfort and dignity of the client. This is an important difference. You will need to adjust your mindset when caring for hospice clients. Focus on relieving their pain and making them comfortable, rather than on teaching them to care for themselves.

Family members or friends who are caregivers for the dying person will appreciate your help. You are providing them with a break. This kind of care is sometimes referred to as respite (RES-pit) care. You must be aware of the feelings of family caregivers. Encourage them to take breaks and take care of themselves. However, do not insist that they do so. Many want to do all they can for their loved one during his or her last days. Do observe family caregivers for signs of excessive stress. Report any signs to your supervisor. Your agency may be able to refer them to local support services.

IV
Client Care

11. Maintaining Mobility, Skin, and Comfort

Transfers/Ambulation

One of the most important considerations during client transfers is safety! Follow these safety guidelines:

Falls

- Widen your stance. Bring the client's body close to you to break the fall. Bend your knees and support the client as you lower her to the floor.

- Do not try to reverse or stop a fall. You or the client can suffer worse injuries if you try to stop a fall than if you just break the fall.

- Call for help if a family member is around. Do not attempt to get the client up after the fall unless you are certain the client is not injured. Follow your agency's policies and procedures. Always call your supervisor if you are unsure of what to do.

- If you do help the client up, get her in bed, take vital signs, then report the fall to your supervisor.

Canes, Walkers, and Crutches

- Ensure safety with whichever device is being used.

- Stay near the person, on the weak side.

- Make sure the equipment is in proper condition. It must be sturdy, and it must have rubber tips or wheels on the bottom.

Wheelchairs

- Learn how a wheelchair works. Know how to apply and release the brake and how to operate the footrests. Lock the wheelchair before assisting a client into or out of it. After the transfer, unlock the wheelchair.

- To transfer to or from a wheelchair, use the side or areas of the client's body that can bear weight to support and lift the side or areas that cannot bear weight.

- Make sure the client is safe and comfortable during transfers. Ask the client how you can assist with wheelchairs. Some clients may only want you to bring the chair to the bedside. Others may want you to be more involved.

- If the client needs to be moved back in the wheelchair, go to the back of the chair. Reach forward and down under the client's arms. Ask the client to place his feet on the ground and push up. Pull the client up in the chair while the client pushes.

Mechanical Lifts

- You may assist the client with many types of transfers using the mechanical or hydraulic lift if you are trained to do so.

- Lifts help prevent injury to you and the client. Never use equipment you have not been trained to use. You or your client could get hurt if you use lifting equipment improperly.

- There are many different types of mechanical lifts. You must be trained on the specific lift you will be using.

Assisting a client to a dangling position

Before a client who has been lying down stands up, she should dangle. To dangle means to sit up with the feet over the side of the bed to regain balance.

1   Wash your hands.

2   Explain the procedure to the client. Speak clearly, slowly, and directly. Maintain face-to-face contact whenever possible.

3   Provide privacy if the client desires it.

4   If the bed is adjustable, adjust bed to lowest position. If bed is movable, lock bed wheels.

5   Raise the head of the bed to a sitting position.

6   Place one arm under the client's shoulder blades. Place the other arm under the client's thighs.

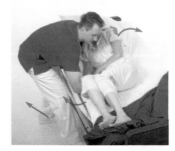

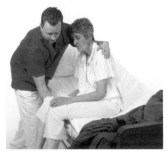

7   On the count of three, slowly turn client into sitting position with legs dangling over side of bed.

8   Ask client to hold onto edge of mattress with both hands. Assist him or her to put on nonskid slippers or shoes.

9   Have client dangle as long as ordered. Stay with the client at all times. Check for dizziness. If client feels dizzy or faint, help her lie down again. Report this to your supervisor.

10 Take vital signs as ordered.

11 Remove slippers or shoes.

12 Gently assist client back into bed. Place one arm around client's shoulders. Place the other under client's knees. Slowly swing client's legs onto bed.

13 Make sure client is comfortable. Remove privacy measures. If you raised an adjustable bed, return it to its proper position.

14 Wash your hands.

15 Document the procedure and your observations. How did the client tolerate sitting up? Did the client become dizzy?

Helping a client sit up using the arm lock

1   Wash your hands.

2   Explain the procedure to the client. Speak clearly, slowly, and directly. Maintain face-to-face contact whenever possible.

3   Provide privacy if the client desires it.

4   If the bed is adjustable, adjust bed to lowest position. If bed is movable, lock bed wheels.

5   Stand facing the head of the bed, with your legs about 12 inches apart and your knees bent. The foot that is further from the bed should be slightly ahead of the other foot.

6   Place your arm under the client's armpit and grasp the client's shoulder. Have the client grasp your shoulder in the same manner. This hold is called the arm lock or lock arm.

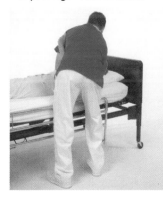

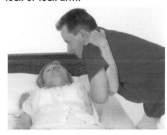

7   Reach under the client's head and place your other hand on the client's far shoulder. Have the client bend her knees. Bend your knees.

8   At the count of three, rock yourself backward and pull the client to a

sitting position. Use pillows or a bed rest to support the client in the sitting position.

9 Check the client for dizziness or weakness.

10 If you raised an adjustable bed, return it to its proper position.

11 Wash your hands.

12 Document the procedure and any observations. Was the client able to help at all? Did the client become dizzy?

Helping a client stand up

1 Wash your hands.

2 Explain the procedure to the client. Speak clearly, slowly, and directly. Maintain face-to-face contact whenever possible.

3 Provide privacy if the client desires it.

4 If the bed is adjustable, adjust bed to lowest position. If bed is movable, lock bed wheels.

5 Assist the client to a dangling position.

6 Put nonskid footwear on client.

7 If the client is able, have her place her hands on the edge of the bed and push to standing, while you stay nearby to steady her or offer support if needed.

8 Always allow your client to do whatever she is able to do for herself. If the client is not able to stand without help, place one foot between the client's feet. If the client has a weak knee, brace it against your knee.

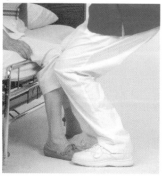

9 Have the client place her stronger leg directly under herself.

10 Bending your knees and leaning forward, put both arms around the client's waist and hold her close to your center of gravity.

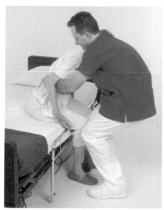

11 Tell the client to lean forward, push down on the bed with her hands, and stand, on the count of three. When you start to count, begin to rock. At three, rock your weight onto your back foot and assist the client to a standing position.

12 Check the client for dizziness before you allow her to stand alone.

13 Wash your hands.

14 Document the procedure and any observations. How did the client tolerate standing? How much help did you offer?

Using a transfer belt to assist with ambulation

A transfer belt, or gait belt, is used to assist clients who are able to walk but are weak, unsteady, or uncoordinated. The belt is made of canvas or other heavy material and fits around the client's waist outside the clothing. The transfer belt is a safety device that gives you something firm to hold on to. When placing the belt on a client, leave enough room to insert two fingers into the belt.

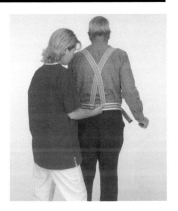

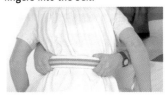

1 Wash your hands.

2 Explain the procedure to the client. Speak clearly, slowly, and directly. Maintain face-to-face contact whenever possible.

3 Provide privacy if the client desires it.

4 If the bed is adjustable, adjust bed to lowest position. If bed is movable, lock bed wheels.

5 Place the belt around the client's waist. Always apply the belt over clothing. Never place it next to skin.

6 Put nonskid footwear on client.

7 Help the client stand up. Observe the client for strength and coordination.

8 Stand behind and to the side of the client as you hold on to the belt. If the client has a weaker side, stand on that side. Use the hand that is not holding the belt to offer support to the client on the weak side.

9 Observe the client's strength while you walk together. Provide a chair if the client becomes dizzy or fatigued.

10 Return the client to the bed or chair and be sure he is comfortable. If you raised an adjustable bed, be sure to return it to the proper position.

11 Wash your hands.

12 Document the procedure and your observations. How far did the client walk? How did the client appear or say he felt while walking? How much help did you give?

Assisting with ambulation for a client who uses a cane, walker, or crutches

1 Wash your hands.

2 Explain the procedure to the client. Speak clearly, slowly, and directly. Maintain face-to-face contact whenever possible.

3 Provide privacy if the client desires it.

4 If the bed is adjustable, adjust bed to lowest position. If bed is movable, lock bed wheels.

5 Fasten the transfer belt around the client's waist.

6 Put nonskid footwear on client.

7 Assist the client to a standing position.

8   Help as needed with ambulation.

a. **Cane**. Client places cane about 12 inches in front of his stronger leg. He brings weaker leg even with cane. He then brings stronger leg forward slightly ahead of cane. Repeat.

b. **Walker**. Client picks up or rolls the walker. He places it about 12 inches in front of him. All four feet or wheels of the walker should be on the ground before client steps forward to the walker. The walker should not be moved again until the client has moved both feet forward and is steady. The client should never put his feet ahead of the walker.

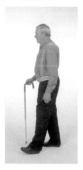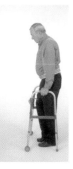

c. **Crutches**. Client should be fitted for crutches and taught to use them correctly by a physical therapist or nurse. The client may use the crutches several different ways. It depends on what his weakness is.

No matter how they are used, weight should be on the client's hands and arms, not on the underarm area.

9   Walk slightly behind the client, on the weak side if the client has one. Hold the transfer belt unless you think the client is steady on his own.

10 Watch for obstacles in the client's path. Encourage the client to look ahead, not down at his feet.

11 Encourage the client to rest if he is tired. When a client is tired, it increases the chance of a fall. Let the client set the pace. Discuss how far he plans to go based on the care plan.

12 After ambulation, remove the transfer belt. Settle the client back into a safe and comfortable position. If you raised an adjustable bed, be sure to return it to the proper position.

13 Wash your hands.

14 Document the procedure and your observations. How did the client feel or appear while walking? How far did the client walk? How much help did the client need?

Helping a client move from a bed to a chair

Equipment: robe and nonskid footwear, transfer belt, chair or wheelchair, sheet or blanket

1   Wash your hands.

2   Explain the procedure to the client. Speak clearly, slowly, and directly. Maintain face-to-face contact whenever possible.

3   Provide privacy if the client desires it. Check the area to be certain it is uncluttered and safe.

4   Assist the client to the dangling position. Put on nonskid footwear.

5   Place the chair or wheelchair at the side of the bed on the client's stronger side. The chair should be at an angle slightly facing the client. If using a wheelchair, lock the brakes and raise or remove the foot and leg rests so they are not in the way. Cover plastic seats with a bath blanket or a soft pillow.

6 Help the client stand up.

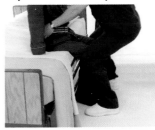

7 Tell the client to take small steps in the direction of the chair while turning his back toward the chair. If more assistance is needed, have the client pivot on the foot that is farthest away from the chair. Always allow the client to do all he can for himself.

8 Have the client use one arm to grasp the arm of the chair. When the chair is touching the back of the client's legs, help the client lower himself into the chair.

9 If using a wheelchair, lower the footrests and help the client place his feet on them. Check that the client is in good alignment. Place a lap robe, folded blanket, or sheet over the lap as appropriate.

10 Wash your hands.

11 Document the procedure and your observations. How did the client feel or appear during the transfer? How much assistance was required?

Helping a client transfer using a slide board

1 Follow steps 1 through 5 of the procedure for helping a client move from a bed to a chair.

2 Have the client lean away from transfer side to take the weight off her thigh. Place one end of the sliding board under the buttocks and thigh. Take care not to pinch the client's skin between the bed and the board. Place the other end of the sliding board on the surface to which the client is transferring.

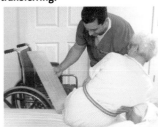

3 If the client is able, have her push up with her hands and scoot herself across the board. Stay close so you can provide support if needed. Always allow the client to do all she can for herself.

4 If the client needs assistance, stand in front of her and put your

knees in front and a little to the outside of her knees to keep them from buckling during the transfer. Make sure your back is straight.

5 Get as close to the client as possible and have her lean into you as you grasp the transfer belt from behind. Lean back with your knees bent. Using your legs rather than your back, pull the client up slightly and toward you to help her scoot across the board.

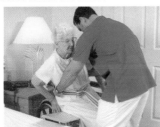

6 Complete the transfer in two or three lifting and scooting movements. Never drag the client across the board. Friction from the client's skin dragging across the slide board can cause skin breakdown that can lead to pressure sores.

7 After the client is safely transferred, remove the sliding board. Make sure the client is positioned safely and comfortably.

8 Wash your hands.

9 Document the procedure and any observations. How did the client feel or appear during the transfer? How much assistance was required?

Transferring a client using a mechanical lift

This is a basic procedure for transferring someone using a mechanical lift. Ask someone to help you before starting.

Equipment: wheelchair or chair, lifting partner, if available, mechanical or hydraulic lift

1 Wash your hands.

2 Explain the procedure to the client. Speak clearly, slowly, and directly. Maintain face-to-face contact whenever possible.

3 Provide privacy if the client desires it.

4 If bed is movable, lock bed wheels.

5 Position wheelchair next to bed. Lock brakes.

6 Help the client turn to one side of the bed. Position the sling under the client, with the edge next to the client's back fanfolded if necessary, and the bottom of the sling even with the client's knees. Help the client roll back to the middle of the bed. Spread out the fanfolded edge of the sling.

7 Roll the mechanical lift to bedside. Make sure the base is opened to its widest point. Push the base of the lift under the bed.

8 Position the overhead bar directly over the client.

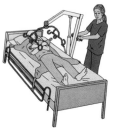

9 With the client lying on his back, attach one set of straps to each side of the sling, and one set of straps to the overhead bar. If available, have a lifting partner support the client at the head, shoulders, and knees while being lifted. The client's arms should be folded across his chest. If the device has "S" hooks, they should face away from client. Make sure all straps are connected properly.

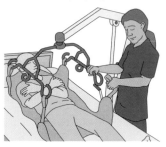

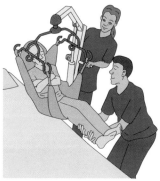

10 Following manufacturer's instructions, raise the client two inches above the bed. Pause a moment for the client to gain his balance.

11 If available, a lifting partner can help support and guide the client's body. You can then roll the lift so

that the client is positioned over the chair or wheelchair.

12 Slowly lower the client into the chair or wheelchair. Push down gently on the client's knees to help the client into a sitting position.

13 Undo the straps from the overhead bar. Leave the sling in place for transfer back to bed.

14 Be sure the client is seated comfortably and correctly in the chair or wheelchair.

15 Wash your hands.

16 Document the procedure and any observations. How did the client tolerate the transfer? Were there any problems during the transfer? Did the equipment operate properly?

Positioning

Clients who spend a lot of time in bed often need help getting into comfortable positions. They also need to change positions periodically to avoid muscle stiffness and skin breakdown or pressure sores. Bed-bound clients should be repositioned every two hours. Document the position and time every time there is a change.

Following are the five basic body positions:

1 Supine

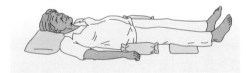

2 Lateral/Side

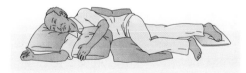

3 Prone

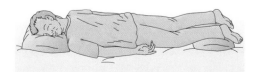

4 Fowler's

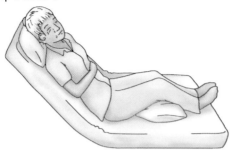

5 Sims'

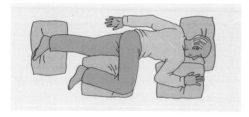

Clients who are confined to bed need to maintain good body alignment. This promotes recovery and prevents injury to muscles and joints. The following guidelines help clients maintain good alignment and make progress when they can get out of bed.

Observe principles of alignment. Remember that proper alignment is based on straight lines. The spine should lie in a straight line. Pillows or rolled or folded blankets may be needed to support the small of the back and raise the knees or head in the supine position. They can support the head and one leg in the lateral position.

Keep body parts in natural positions. In a natural hand position, the fingers are slightly curled. Use a rolled washcloth, gauze bandage, or a rubber ball inside the palm to support the fingers in this position. Use footboards to keep covers from resting on feet in the supine position.

Prevent external rotation of hips. When legs and hips are allowed to turn outward during prolonged bed rest, hip contractures can result. A

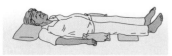

trochanter (troh-KAN-ter) roll is a rolled blanket or towel that is tucked alongside the hip and thigh to prevent the leg from turning outward.

Change positions frequently to prevent muscle stiffness and pressure sores. Every two hours is usually adequate. Which positions a client uses will depend on the client's condition and preference. Check the skin every time you reposition a client. Immobility reduces the amount of oxygen-carrying blood that circulates to the skin. Clients who have restricted mobility have increased risk of skin deterioration at pressure points.

GUIDELINES: POSITIONING

- Have plenty of pillows available to provide support in the various positions.

- Use positioning devices (such as backrests, bed cradles and tables, footboards, and handrolls).

- Give back rubs for comfort and relaxation.

- Change positions frequently (every two hours) and as directed in the care plan.

- Always maintain the client's body alignment.

For more information on using positioning devices for comfort, refer to the "Comfort Measures" section.

Range of Motion Exercises

Exercise helps people regain strength and mobility. It prevents disabilities from developing. People who are in bed for long periods of time are more likely to develop contractures. A contracture is the permanent and often very painful stiffening of a joint and muscle. Contractures are generally caused by immobility and result in a loss of ability. Range of motion (ROM) exercises are exercises that put a particular joint through its full arc of motion. The purpose of ROM exercises is to decrease or prevent contractures, improve strength, and increase circulation.

Passive range of motion (PROM) exercises are used when clients are not able to move on their own. When assisting with PROM exercises, support the client's joints and move them through the range of motion. Active range of motion (AROM) exercises are performed by a client himself. Your role in AROM exercises is to encourage the client. Active assisted range of motion (AAROM) exercises are performed by the client with some assistance and support from you.

You will not perform ROM exercises without a specific order from a doctor, nurse, or physical therapist. When performing ROM exercises, begin at the client's head and work down the body. Stop the motion if the client complains of pain. These exercises are specific for each body area. They include the following movements:

- Abduction: moving a body part away from the body
- Adduction: moving a body part toward the body
- Dorsiflexion: bending backward
- Rotation: turning a joint
- Extension: straightening a body part
- Flexion: bending a body part
- Pronation: turning downward
- Supination: turning upward

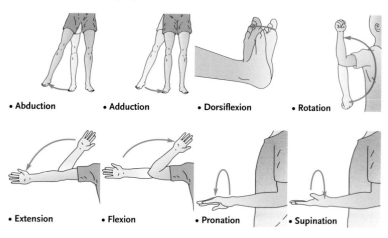

• Abduction   • Adduction   • Dorsiflexion   • Rotation

• Extension   • Flexion   • Pronation   • Supination

Assisting with passive range of motion exercises

1   Wash your hands.

2   Explain the procedure to the client. Speak clearly, slowly, and directly. Maintain face-to-face contact whenever possible.

3   Provide privacy if the client desires it.

4   If the bed is adjustable, adjust bed to a safe working level, usually waist high. If bed is movable, lock bed wheels.

5   Position the client supine on the bed. Position the body in good alignment.

6   Shoulder
Support the client's arm at the elbow and wrist while performing ROM for the shoulder. Place one hand above the elbow and the other hand around the wrist. Move the arm upward so that the upper arm is aligned with the side of the head (forward flexion). Move the arm downward to the side (extension). Return arm to side. Bring the arm sideways away from the body to above the head (abduction) and back down to midline (adduction). Bend the elbow and position it at the same level as the shoulder. Move the forearm down toward the body (internal rotation). Now move the

forearm toward the head (external rotation).

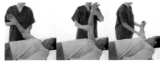

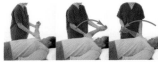

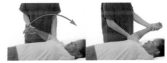

7 Elbow

Hold the client's wrist with one hand, the elbow with the other hand. Bend the elbow so that the hand touches the shoulder on that same side (flexion). Straighten the arm (extension). Exercise the forearm by moving it so the palm is facing downward (pronation) and then is facing upward (supination).

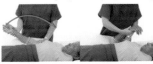

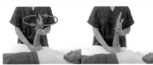

8 Wrist

Hold the wrist with one hand and use the fingers of the other hand to help the joint through the motions. Bend the hand down (flexion); bend the hand backwards (extension). Turn the hand in the direction of the thumb (radial flexion); turn the hand in the direction of the little finger (ulnar flexion).

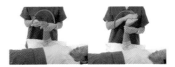

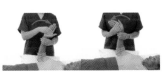

9 Thumb

Move the thumb away from the index finger (abduction). Move the thumb back next to the index finger (adduction). Touch each fingertip with the thumb (opposition). Bend thumb into the palm (flexion) and out to the side (extension).

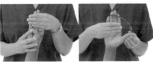

10 Fingers

Make the hand into a fist (flexion). Straighten out the fist (extension). Spread the fingers and the thumb far apart from each other (abduction). Bring the fingers next to each other (adduction).

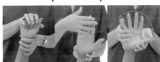

11 Hip

Support the leg by placing one hand under the knee and one under the ankle. Straighten the leg and raise it gently upward. Move the leg away from the other leg (abduction). Move the leg toward the other leg (adduction). Gently turn the leg inward (internal rotation), then turn the leg outward (external rotation).

12 Knees

Bend the leg at the knee (flexion). Straighten the leg (extension).

13 Ankles

Bend the foot up toward the leg (dorsiflexion). Turn the foot down away from the leg (plantar flexion). Turn the inside of the foot inward toward the body (supination) and the sole of the foot so that it faces away from the body (pronation).

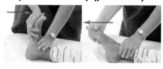

14 Toes

Curl and straighten the toes (flexion and extension). Gently spread the toes apart (abduction).

15 Return the client to a comfortable resting position and cover as appropriate.

16 Wash your hands.

17 Document the procedure. Note any decrease in range of motion or any pain experienced by the client. Notify the supervisor or the physical therapist if you find increased stiffness or physical resistance. Resistance may be a sign that a contracture is developing.

Skin Care

Clients who have restricted mobility have increased risk of skin deterioration at pressure points. Pressure points are areas of the body that bear much of the body weight. Pressure points are mainly located at bony prominences. Bony prominences are areas of the body where the bone lies close to the skin. These areas include elbows, shoulder blades, tailbone, hip bones, ankles, heels, and the back of the neck and head.

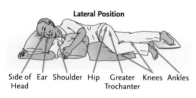

Lateral Position

Side of Head   Ear   Shoulder   Hip   Greater Trochanter   Knees   Ankles

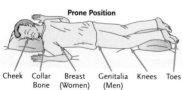

Prone Position

Cheek   Collar Bone   Breast (Women)   Genitalia (Men)   Knees   Toes

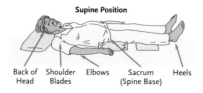

Supine Position

Back of Head   Shoulder Blades   Elbows   Sacrum (Spine Base)   Heels

Other areas at risk are the ears, the area under the breasts, and the scrotum. The pressure on these areas reduces circulation, decreasing the amount of oxygen the cells receive. Warmth and moisture also contribute to skin breakdown. Once the surface of the skin is weakened, pathogens can invade and cause infection. When infection occurs, the healing process slows down.

When the skin begins to break down, it becomes pale, white or a reddened color. Darker skin may appear purple. The client may also complain of tingling or burning in the area. This discoloration does not go away, even when the client's position is changed. If pressure is allowed to continue, the area will further deteriorate, or break down. The resulting wound is called a pressure sore, bed sore, or decubitus ulcer (dee-KYOO-bi-tus). Once a pressure sore forms, it can get bigger, deeper, and infected. Pressure sores are painful and are difficult to heal. Prevention is very important.

CLIENT'S SKIN: OBSERVING AND REPORTING

- pale, white, reddened, or purple areas, or blistered or bruised areas on the skin
- complaints of tingling, warmth, or burning of the skin
- dry or flaking skin
- itching or scratching
- rash or any skin discoloration
- swelling
- blisters
- fluid or blood draining from skin
- broken skin
- wounds or ulcers on the skin
- changes in an existing wound or ulcer (size, depth, drainage, color, odor)
- redness or broken skin between toes or around toenails

GUIDELINES: BASIC SKIN CARE

- Report changes you observe in a client's skin.
- Provide regular care for skin to keep it clean and dry. When complete baths are not given or taken every day, check the client's skin and provide skin care daily.
- Reposition immobile clients frequently (at least every two hours).
- Provide frequent and thorough skin care for incontinent clients. Change clothing and linens often as well.
- Avoid scratching or irritating the skin in any way. Report to your supervisor if a client wears shoes or slippers that cause blisters or sores.
- Massage the skin frequently, using light, circular strokes to increase circulation. Use little or no pressure on bony areas. Do not massage a white, red, or purple area or put any pressure on it. Massage the healthy skin and tissue surrounding the area.

For clients who are confined to bed or who spend a great deal of time in bed or in a certain position, remember the following:

- Keep the bottom sheet tight and free from wrinkles and the bed free from crumbs.

- Avoid pulling the client across sheets during transfers or repositioning. Dragging the client's skin across the surface of the sheet causes shearing, or pressure, when the surfaces rub against each other.

- Place a sheepskin, chamois skin, or bed pad under the back and buttocks to absorb moisture. This also protects the skin from irritating bed linens.

- Relieve pressure under bony prominences. Place foam rubber or sheepskin pads under them. Heel and elbow protectors that are made of foam and sheepskin are available.

- A bed or chair can be made softer with flotation pads or an egg crate mattress.

- Use a bed cradle to keep top sheets from rubbing the client's skin. A bed cradle is made of metal or from a cardboard box.

- Reposition clients seated in chairs or wheelchairs frequently.

Comfort Measures

There are several things you can do to provide for the comfort and safety of your client in and around the bed. Many positioning devices are available to help make clients more comfortable. Some can be inexpensively made in the client's home. Check with your supervisor on the use of positioning devices for each client.

GUIDELINES: USING POSITIONING DEVICES

- Backrests can be made of pillows, cardboard or wood covered by pillows, or special wedge-shaped foam pillows.

- Bed cradles are used to keep the bed covers from pushing down on client's feet. Metal frames that work like a tent when the bed covers are over them can be purchased. A cardboard box can be used as a bed cradle by placing the client's feet inside the box underneath the covers. The box should be at least two inches above the toes.

- Bed tables are available commercially. You can also make one by cutting openings in each of the longer sides of a sturdy cardboard box.

- Draw sheets may be placed under a client to help move clients who are unable to assist with turning in bed, lifting, or moving up in bed. Draw sheets also help prevent skin damage that can be caused by shearing. A regular bed sheet folded in half can be used as a draw sheet.

- Foot boards are padded boards placed against the client's feet to keep them flexed and prevent footdrop. Rolled blankets or pillows can also be used as foot boards.

- Hand rolls keep the fingers from curling tightly. A rolled washcloth, gauze bandage, or a rubber ball placed inside the palm may be used to keep the hand in a natural position.

A back rub can help relax your client and make her more comfortable. Back rubs increase circulation, too. Back rubs are often given after baths.

Giving a back rub

Equipment: cotton blanket or towel, lotion, gloves if client's skin is broken

1   Wash your hands.

2   Explain the procedure to the client. Speak clearly, slowly, and directly. Maintain face-to-face contact whenever possible.

3   Provide privacy if the client desires it.

4   If the bed is adjustable, adjust bed to a safe working level, usually waist high. Lower the head of the bed until it is flat. If bed is movable, lock bed wheels.

5   Have the client lie in a prone position. If this is uncomfortable, have the client lie on his side. Cover the client with a cotton blanket, then fold back the bed covers. Expose the client's back to the top of the buttocks. If the client is positioned on his side, place the towel on the bed along the length of his back. Back rubs can also be given with the client sitting up.

6   Warm the lotion bottle in warm water for five minutes. Run your hands under warm water to warm them. Pour the lotion on your hands. Rub them together to spread it. Warn the client that the lotion may still feel cool. Always put the lotion on your hands rather than directly on the client's skin.

7   Place your hands on each side of the upper part of the buttocks. Make long, smooth upward strokes with both hands along each side of the spine, up to the shoulders. Circle your hands outward. Then move back along the outer edges of the back. At the buttocks, make another circle and move your hands back up to the shoulders. Without taking your hands from the client's skin, repeat this motion for three to five minutes.

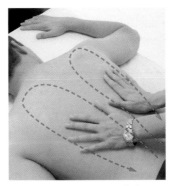

8   Make kneading motions with the first two fingers and thumb of each hand. Place them at the base of the spine. Move upward together along each side of the spine, applying gen-

tle downward pressure with the fingers and thumbs. Follow the same direction as with the long smooth strokes, circling at shoulders and buttocks.

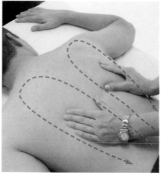

9   Gently massage bony areas (spine, shoulder blades, hip bones) with circular motions of your fingertips. Gentle massage stimulates circulation and helps prevent skin damage. However, if any of these areas are red, massage around them rather than on them. The redness indicates that the skin is already irritated and fragile.

10   Let your client know when you are almost through. Finish with some long smooth strokes, like the ones you used at the beginning of the massage.

11   Dry the back if extra lotion remains on it. If appropriate, apply powder to the back to allow better movement against the sheets.

12   Remove the cotton blanket and towel.

13   Assist the client with getting dressed.

14   Help the client into a comfortable position. If you raised an adjustable bed, be sure to return it to its lowest position.

15   Store the lotion and put dirty linens in the hamper.

16   Wash your hands.

17   Document the procedure and your observations. Did the client appear comfortable during the back rub? Did you observe any discolored areas or broken skin?

12. Personal Care Procedures

If you are already a CNA or HHA, you have previously learned personal care skills. This section will serve as a review of the basic skills and procedures most often provided for clients in their homes. Clients should be encouraged to do as much of the care by themselves as possible. This promotes independence.

Personal care includes such activities as bathing, perineal care (care of the area around and between the genitals and anus), mouth care, shampooing and combing the hair, nail care, shaving, dressing, and changing bed linens.

Before you begin any task, explain to the client exactly what you will be doing. Ask if he or she would like to use the bathroom or bedpan first. Provide the client with privacy. Let him or her make as many decisions as possible about when, where, and how a procedure will be done. This promotes dignity and independence. During the procedure, if the client appears tired, stop and take a short rest. After care, always ask if the client would like anything else.

PERSONAL CARE: OBSERVING AND REPORTING

- skin, mobility, flexibility, comfort level, and ability to perform ADLs
- client complaints
- mental and emotional state

Bathing

Bathing promotes good health and well-being. It removes perspiration, dirt, oil, and dead skin cells that collect on the skin. The bed bath is an excellent time for moving arms and legs and increasing circulation. Many agencies have rules against HHAs helping clients into the bathtub. These rules are for the client's safety as well as the home health aide's. Follow your agency's policies and procedures.

GUIDELINES: BATHING

- The face, hands, axillae (AK-sil-eye, or underarms), and perineum should be washed every day. A complete bath or shower can be taken every other day or even less frequently.

- Older skin produces less perspiration and oil. Elderly people whose skin is dry and fragile should bathe only once or twice a week.

- Before any bathing task, make sure the room is warm enough.

- Remove any loose rugs that do not have slip-resistant, rubber backings.

- Be familiar with available safety and assistive devices.

- Never leave an elderly person or young child alone in the bathtub.

- Never use bath oils.

Helping the client transfer to the bathtub

Equipment: chair, transfer belt (if appropriate), shirt or robe to wear under transfer belt, slide board (if appropriate), tub or shower chair, bath supplies (listed in next procedure), gloves

1 Wash your hands.

2 Explain the procedure to the client. Speak clearly, slowly, and directly. Maintain face-to-face contact whenever possible.

3 Help the client to the bathroom.

4 Provide privacy for the client.

5 Seat the client in a chair facing the bathtub and centered between the grab bars. If using a wheelchair, lock brakes and raise footrests.

6 Ask the client to place one leg at a time over the sides of the tub.

7 Have client hold onto the grab bars or the edge of the tub to

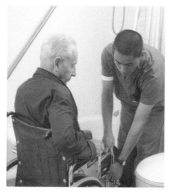

bring himself to a sitting position on the edge of the tub. A slide board may also be used to help the client move from the chair to the tub.

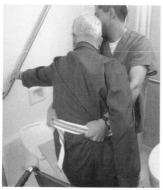

8   Help the client lower himself into the tub or onto the tub chair while holding onto the edge of the tub

or grab bars. If necessary, assist by holding him around the waist or by having him wear a transfer belt. If using a transfer belt to get in and out of the tub, the client will need to wear a shirt or robe while transferring, so the belt is not placed directly against his skin.

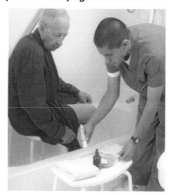

9   Reverse this procedure to help the client out of the tub when the bath is over. If the client has trouble getting out of the tub, help him to his hands and knees. From that position, he can use the grab bar or the edge of the tub to help pull himself up. You can also help by putting the transfer belt back on the client (over a robe).

10 Wash your hands.

11 Document the procedure and your observations.

Helping the ambulatory client take a shower or tub bath

Equipment: two bath towels, washcloth, soap or other cleanser, bath thermometer (if available), rubber bath mat, tub or shower chair (if appropriate), table for bath supplies and bell (for clients who bathe without assistance), non-skid bath rug, deodorant, lotion and other toiletries, clean clothes or a robe, shoes or non-skid slippers, gloves

1   Wash your hands.

2   Explain the procedure to the client. Speak clearly, slowly, and directly. Maintain face-to-face contact whenever possible.

3   Clean tub or shower if necessary. Place rubber mat on tub or shower floor. Set up tub or shower chair. Place skid-resistant bath rug on the floor next to the tub or shower.

4   Provide privacy for the client.

5   Wash your hands again. Put on gloves if client has broken skin.

6   Fill the tub with warm water (105° F to 110° F on the bath thermometer, or test the water on the inside of your wrist to see if it is comfortable) or adjust the shower water temperature. Have the client test water temperature to see if it is comfortable.

7   Ask the client to undress, and assist as needed. Help client transfer to bathtub or step in the shower.

8   If the care plan allows you to leave the client to bathe alone, place the bathing supplies on a small table within the client's reach. Place a bell or other signal on the table. Tell the client to signal when you are needed. Ask the client not to add more hot or warm water and not to remain in the tub more than 20 minutes. Do not lock the bathroom door. Check on your client every five minutes. If the client is weak, remain in the bathroom. Otherwise, you can make the client's bed while he is in the tub.

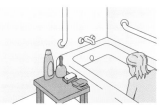

9   For a shower, stay with the client and assist with washing hard-to-reach areas. Observe for signs of fatigue.

10 If the client needs more assistance in the bath or shower, help him wash himself. Always wash from clean areas to dirty areas, so you do not spread dirt into areas that have already been washed. Make sure all soap is rinsed off so the client's skin does not become dry or irritated.

11 Assist the client with shampooing hair, if necessary. Make sure all shampoo is rinsed out of hair.

12 When the bath or shower is finished, help the client get out of the tub. Wrap him in a towel. Have the client sit in a chair or on the toilet seat, and provide him with another towel for drying himself. Offer assistance in drying hard-to-reach places. The client may need help applying powder, deodorant, or lotion. If necessary, help the client get dressed.

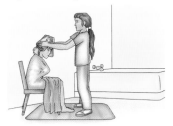

13 If your client is tired after the bath or shower, help him back to the bed. Other personal care, such as mouth care, can be done later or while the client is in bed.

14 Clean the tub and place soiled laundry (towels, washcloths, dirty clothes) in the laundry hamper.

15 Wash your hands.

16 Put away supplies.

17 Document the procedure and your observations. Did you observe any redness or whiteness on the skin? Was there any broken skin? How did the client tolerate bathing or showering? Has there been a change in the client's abilities since the last bath or shower?

Assisting with a bed bath

Equipment: basin, bath thermometer (if available), soap, two washcloths, two or three towels, orangewood stick or nail brush (if available), lotion, deodorant, soft cotton blanket or a large towel, clean clothes, clean bed linens, gloves

1   Wash your hands.

2   Explain the procedure to the client. Speak clearly, slowly, and directly. Maintain face-to-face contact whenever possible.

3   Provide privacy for the client. Be sure the room is a comfortable temperature and there are no drafts.

4   If the bed is adjustable, adjust bed to a safe working level, usually waist high. If the bed is movable, lock bed wheels.

5   Ask client to remove glasses and jewelry and put them in a safe place. Offer to bring bedpan or urinal for the client to use before the bath.

6   Place a soft cotton blanket or towel over client and ask him to hold on to it as you remove the top sheet and blanket. Check the sheets for spills or body discharges.

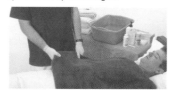

7   Fill the basin with warm water and check the temperature with a bath thermometer or against the inside of your wrist. Water temperature should be between 105° F and 110° F on a thermometer. Allow the client to check the temperature to see if it is adequate. During the bath, change the water when it becomes too cool, soapy, or dirty.

8   If the client has open wounds or broken skin, put on gloves.

9   Ask and assist the client to participate in washing.

10   Uncover only one part of the body at a time. Place a towel under the body part being washed.

11   Wash, rinse, and dry one part of the body at a time. Start at the head, work down, and complete the front first. Fold the washcloth over your hand like a mitt and hold it in place with the thumb.

Eyes and Face: Wash face with wet washcloth (no soap). Begin with the eye farther away from you and wash inner aspect to outer aspect. Use a different area of the washcloth for each eye. Wash the face from the middle outward using firm but gentle strokes. Wash the neck and ears and behind the ears. Rinse and pat dry.

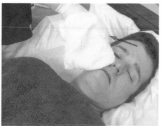

Arms: Remove the client's top clothing, and cover him with a bath blanket or towel. With a soapy washcloth, wash the upper arm and the underarm. Use long strokes from the shoulder down to the elbow. Rinse and pat dry. Wash the elbow. Wash, rinse, and dry from the elbow down to the wrist.

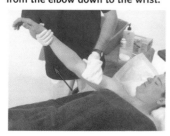

Wash the hand in a basin: Clean under the nails with an orangewood stick or nail brush, if available. Rinse and pat dry. Provide nail care if it has been assigned to you. Do not provide nail care for diabetic clients. Repeat for the other arm and hand. Put lotion on the client's elbows and hands if ordered.

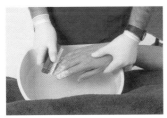

Chest: Place the towel again across the client's chest. Pull the blanket down to the waist. Lift the towel only enough to wash the chest, rinse it, and pat dry. For a female client, wash, rinse, and dry breasts and under breasts. Check the skin in this area for signs of irritation and chafing.

Abdomen: Fold the cotton blanket down so that it still covers the pubic area. Wash the abdomen, rinse, and pat dry. If the client has an ostomy (AH-stoh-mee), or opening in the abdomen for getting rid of body wastes, provide skin care around the opening. Cover with the towel. Pull the cotton blanket up to the client's chin. Remove the towel.

Legs: Expose one leg and place a towel under it. Wash the thigh. Use long, downward strokes. Rinse and pat dry. Do the same from the knee to the ankle. Place another towel under the foot and transfer the basin to the towel. Place the foot into the basin. Wash the foot and between the toes. Rinse foot and pat dry, making sure the area between toes is dry. Perform nail care only if it has been assigned. Do not perform nail care for a diabetic client. Never clip a client's toenails.

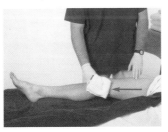

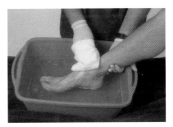

Apply lotion to the foot if ordered, especially at the heels. Repeat steps for the other leg and foot.

Back: Help the client move to the center of the bed then turn onto his side so his back is facing you. If the bed has rails, raise the rail on the opposite side for safety. Fold the cotton blanket away from the back. Place a towel lengthwise next to the back. Wash the back, neck, and buttocks with long, downward strokes. Rinse and pat dry. Apply lotion if ordered.

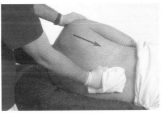

12 Place the towel under the buttocks and upper thighs. Help the client turn onto his back. Ask the client if he is able to complete the bath by washing the perineal area. If the client is able to do this, place a basin of clean, warm water within reach, along with a washcloth and towel. Leave the room if the client would like privacy. If the client has a urinary catheter in place, remind him or her not to pull it.

13 If the client is unable to provide perineal care, you must do so. Put on gloves (if you have not already done so) before washing perineal area. Provide privacy at all times.

14 **For a female client**: Wash the perineum with soap and water from front to back, using single strokes. Do not wash from the back to the

front. This may cause infection. Use a clean area of the washcloth or a clean washcloth for each stroke. First wipe the center of the perineum, then each side. Then spread the labia majora (LAY-bee-a ma-JOHR-a), the outside folds of perineal skin that protect the urinary meatus and the vaginal opening. Wipe from front to back on each side. Wipe down the middle. Rinse the area in the same way. Dry entire perineal area. Move from front to back. Use a blotting motion with towel. Ask the client to turn on her side. Wash, rinse, and dry buttocks and anal area. Clean the anal area without contaminating the perineal area.

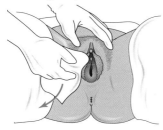

For a male client: If the client is uncircumcised, retract the foreskin first. Gently push skin towards the base of penis. Hold the penis by the shaft. Wash in a circular motion from the tip down to the base. Rinse the penis. Then wash the scrotum and groin. The groin is the area from the pubis (area around the penis and scrotum) to the upper thighs. Rinse and pat dry. If client is uncircumcised, gently return foreskin to normal position. Ask the client to turn on his side. Wash, rinse, and dry buttocks and anal area. Clean the anal area without contaminating the perineal area.

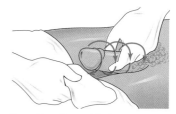

15 Cover the client with the cotton blanket.

16 Place soiled washcloths and towels in the hamper or laundry basket. Dispose of the dirty bath water in the toilet. Discard gloves into a trash receptacle.

17 If time permits, a bed bath is a good time to give the client a back rub if he wants one.

18 Provide the client with deodorant. Place a towel over the pillow and brush or comb the client's hair. Help the client put on clean clothing and get into a comfortable position with good body alignment. If you raised an adjustable bed, be sure to return it to its lowest position.

19 If the client uses a signaling device, place it within reach. Take the bath supplies away, and wash and store everything. Change bed sheets and blanket. Place used bed linens in the hamper or laundry basket.

20 Wash your hands.

21 Document the procedure and your observations. Did you observe any redness or whiteness on the skin? Was there any broken skin? How did the client tolerate bathing? Did the client tell you about any symptoms? Has there been a change in the client's abilities since the last bath?

Grooming

When assisting clients with grooming, always allow the clients to do all they can for themselves. Follow the instructions in the care plan. Some clients have particular ways of grooming themselves. They may have a routine. Some clients may be embarrassed or depressed because they need help with grooming tasks they have performed for themselves all their lives. Be sensitive to this. Be professional, respectful and cheerful while assisting your clients with grooming.

Nail care should only be provided if it has specifically been assigned. Never cut a client's toenails. In some clients, poor circulation can lead to infection if skin is accidently cut while caring for nails. In a diabetic client, such an infection can lead to a severe wound or even amputation. If you are directed to provide nail care, know exactly what care you need to provide.

Providing fingernail care

Equipment: orangewood stick, emery board, small basin or bowl, lotion, cuticle softener, bath towel, soap, bath thermometer, gloves if client has broken skin

1   Wash your hands.

2   Explain the procedure to the client. Speak clearly, slowly, and directly. Maintain face-to-face contact whenever possible.

3   Provide privacy for the client.

4   If the bed is adjustable, adjust bed to a safe working level, usually waist high. If the bed is movable, lock bed wheels.

5   Put on gloves if the client has any broken skin.

6   If necessary, remove nail polish with a cotton ball soaked with nail polish remover.

7   Fill the basin halfway full with warm water. Test water temperature with the bath thermometer or with your wrist to ensure it is safe. Water temperature should be 105° F. Have client check the water temperature. Adjust if necessary.

8   Soak the client's nails in the water. If you need to soften cuticles to push them back (step 10, below), add a cuticle softener to the water or apply to the cuticles. Soak all

ten fingertips for two to four minutes.

9   Remove hands from water. Wash hands with soapy washcloth. Rinse. Dry the client's hands with a towel, including between the fingers. Remove the hand basin.

10 Place the client's hands on the towel. Gently push back the cuticles using the flat end of the orangewood stick or a towel.

11 Use the pointed end of the orangewood stick or a nail brush to remove dirt from under the nails. Wipe orangewood stick on towel after cleaning under each nail. Wash the hands again. Dry them thoroughly.

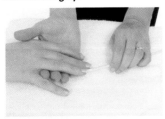

12 Shape fingernails with an emery board or nail file. Apply lotion.

13 Discard the water and clean the basin. Dispose of towels in the laundry hamper and store supplies. If you raised an adjustable

bed, be sure to return it to its lowest position.

14 Wash your hands.

Providing foot care

Equipment: basin, pumice stone (optional), two bath towels, washcloth, lotion, soap, clean socks, bath thermometer, gloves if client has broken skin

1 Wash your hands.

2 Explain the procedure to the client, speaking clearly, slowly, and directly, maintaining face-to-face contact whenever possible.

3 Provide privacy for the client.

4 Put on gloves if the client has any broken skin.

5 Fill the basin halfway with warm water. Test water temperature with the bath thermometer or with your wrist to ensure it is safe. Water temperature should be 105°F. Have the client check the water temperature. Adjust if necessary. Place basin on a bath towel on the floor (if the client is sitting in a chair) or on a towel at the foot of the bed (if the client is in bed).

6 Soak the client's feet for ten minutes. Add warm water to the basin as necessary.

7 Remove one foot from basin. Smooth any rough areas with the pumice stone or a washcloth. Wash entire foot, including between the toes and around nail beds, with a soapy washcloth.

8 Rinse entire foot, including between the toes. Thoroughly dry entire foot, including between the

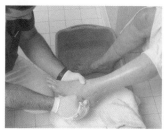

15 Document procedure and any observations.

toes. Apply lotion. Do not attempt any further care of the toenails.

9 Repeat steps 7-8 for other foot.

10 While you are giving foot care, observe the feet for sores, irritated or reddened areas (especially on the heels), any discoloration or darkening on the foot, discoloration of the toes or toenails, swelling, infection, or differences in temperature. Even if another person gives your client foot care, you should still observe for these signs of problems or illness on a regular basis.

11 Assist client to replace socks.

12 Discard the water and clean the basin. Dispose of the towels in the laundry hamper and store supplies.

13 Wash your hands.

14 Document procedure and any observations. Was there any redness, whiteness, or broken or discolored skin? Were there any differences in temperature?

Clients who can get out of bed may have their hair shampooed in the sink, tub, or shower. For clients who cannot get out of bed, special troughs exist for shampooing hair in bed. Troughs fit under the client's head and neck and have a spout or hose that drains the water into a basin at the side of the bed. Your agency should be able to provide this equipment. You may also use a plastic garbage bag formed around a rolled towel.

Shampooing hair

Equipment: shampoo, hair conditioner (if requested), washcloth, pitcher, plastic cup or hand-held shower or sink attachment, chair (for washing hair in sink), large garbage bag or plastic sheet (for washing hair in sink), towel (two towels if washing hair in bed), cotton blanket (for washing hair in bed), waterproof mat (for washing hair in bed), trough or garbage bag and extra towel (for washing hair in bed), catch basin (for washing hair in bed)

1 Wash your hands.

2 Explain the procedure to the client. Speak clearly, slowly, and directly. Maintain face-to-face contact whenever possible.

3 Provide privacy for the client.

4 Position the client and wet the client's hair.

a. ***For washing hair in the sink,*** seat the client in a chair covered with plastic. Use a pillow under the plastic to support the head and neck. Have the client lean her head back toward the sink. Give the client a folded washcloth to hold over her forehead or eyes. Wet hair using a plastic cup or a hand-held sink attachment.

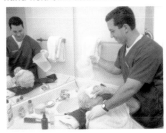

b. ***For washing hair in the tub,*** have the client tilt her head back. Give the client a folded washcloth to hold over her forehead or eyes.

Wet hair using a plastic cup or hand-held shower attachment.

c. ***For washing hair in the shower,*** have the client turn so her back is toward the shower head. Ask the client to tilt her head backwards. Direct the flow of water over the hair to wet it.

d. ***For washing hair in bed,*** arrange the supplies within reach on a nearby table. Remove all pillows, and place the client in a flat position. If bed is adjustable, adjust bed to a safe working level, usually waist high. If the bed is movable, lock bed wheels. Place a waterproof sheet or mat beneath the client's head and shoulders. Cover the client with the cotton blanket, and fold back the top sheet and regular blankets. Place the trough under the client's head, then connect the trough to the catch basin. Using the pitcher, pour enough water on the client's hair to make it thoroughly wet.

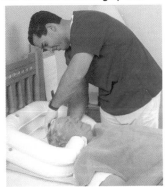

5 Apply a small amount of shampoo to your hands and rub them together. Using both hands, massage the shampoo to a lather in the client's hair. With your fingertips, massage the scalp in a circular motion, from front to back.

6   Rinse the hair in the same way you wet it. Repeat the shampoo, rinse again, and use conditioner if the client wants it. Be sure to rinse the hair thoroughly to prevent the client's scalp from getting dry and itchy.

7   Wrap the client's hair in a towel. If shampooing at the sink, return the client to an upright position. If shampooing in the bath or shower, assist the client from the tub or shower. If shampooing in bed, remove the trough. Using the washcloth or a face towel, wipe water from the head and neck.

8   Remove the hair towel and comb or brush hair (see procedure later in the chapter).

9   Dry hair with a hair dryer on the low setting. Style hair as the client prefers.

10 Wash and store equipment. Put soiled towels and washcloth in the hamper or laundry basket. If you raised an adjustable bed, be sure to return it to its lowest position.

11 Wash your hands.

12 Document the procedure and your observations. How did the client tolerate having her hair washed? Was the client able to help? Have the client's abilities changed since the last time her hair was washed?

Helping a client shave

Equipment: a clean safety, disposable, or electric razor, shaving cream or gel (if using a safety or disposable razor), basin filled with warm water (if using a safety or disposable razor), bath towel, washcloth, mirror, aftershave lotion, gloves

Be sure the client wants you to shave him or help him shave before you begin.

1   Wash your hands.

2   Explain the procedure to the client. Speak clearly, slowly, and directly. Maintain face-to-face contact whenever possible.

3   Provide privacy for the client.

4   Put on gloves. Place the equipment on a table within reach of the client if he will shave himself. If the client is confined to bed, use pillows or a backrest to help him sit up in a comfortable position. If the bed is adjustable, adjust bed to a safe working level, usually waist high. If bed is movable, lock bed wheels. If the client wears dentures, be sure they are in place. Place the towel across the client's chest.

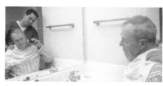

5   If you are using an electric razor, use a small brush to clean it. Do not use an electric razor near any water source, when oxygen is in use, or if the client has a pacemaker. Turn on the razor and shave the face, pulling the skin tight over the mouth and cheeks if necessary to shave more smoothly. Shave the chin and under the chin.

6   If you are using a safety or disposable razor, use a blade that is sharp. A dull blade is hard on the skin. Soften the beard with a warm wet towel on the face for a few minutes before shaving. Lather the face with shaving cream or gel and warm water. Warm water and lather make shaving more comfortable. Shaving in the direction of hair growth is also more comfortable. It will result in a more even shave. Use short strokes on the chin and longer strokes on the cheeks. Rinse the blade frequently in the basin.

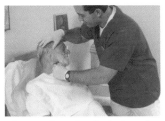

7 When you have finished, rinse the client's face with a warm, wet washcloth or let him use the washcloth himself. Offer a mirror to the client.

8 If the client wants aftershave, moisten your palms with after-shave lotion and pat it onto the client's face.

9 Clean the equipment and store it. Dispose of the used razor blade or disposable razor. Put the towel and washcloth in the hamper or laundry basket. Remove and discard gloves. If you raised an adjustable bed, be sure to return it to its lowest position.

10 Wash your hands.

11 Document the procedure and any observations.

Combing or brushing hair

Equipment: comb, brush, or hair pick, bath towel, mirror, hair care items requested by the client, gloves if client has broken skin on scalp or face

Use hair care products that the client prefers for his or her type of hair.

1 Wash your hands.

2 Explain the procedure to the client. Speak clearly, slowly, and directly. Maintain face-to-face contact whenever possible.

3 Provide privacy for the client.

4 If the client is confined to bed, raise the head of the bed, use a backrest, or use pillows to raise the client's head and shoulders. If the bed is adjustable, adjust bed to a safe working level, usually waist high. If the bed is movable, lock bed wheels. Place the towel under the client's head. If the client is ambulatory, provide a chair. Place the towel around client's shoulders.

5 Put on gloves only if the client has broken skin on the scalp or face.

6 Remove any hairpins, hair ties, and clips.

7 If the hair is tangled, work on the tangles first. Remove tangles by dividing hair into small sections. Hold the lock of hair just above the tangle so you don't pull at the scalp. Gently comb or brush through the tangle. Gently comb out from ends of hair to scalp. If client agrees, you can use a small amount of detangler or leave-in conditioner on the tangle.

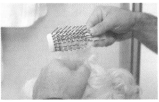

8 Brush two-inch sections of hair at a time. Brush from roots to ends.

9 Each client may prefer a different hairstyle. Style hair in the way the client prefers. Avoid childish hairstyles. Offer a mirror to the client.

10 Remove the towel and shake excess hair in the wastebasket. Place the soiled towel in the hamper. Store supplies. Remove gloves. If you raised an adjustable bed, be sure to return it to its lowest position.

11 Wash your hands.

12 Document the procedure and any observations.

GUIDELINES: HELPING A CLIENT DRESS AND UNDRESS

- Client's preferences should be asked and followed.

- Allow the client to choose clothing for the day. However, check to see if it is clean, appropriate for the weather, and in good condition.

- Encourage the client to dress in regular clothes rather than night-clothes.

- The client should do as much to dress or undress himself as possible.

- Provide privacy.

- Roll or fold socks or stockings so they can be slipped over toes and foot, then unrolled into place.

- Front-fastening bras are easier for clients to manage by themselves.

- If a client has a weakened side due to a stroke or injury, that side is called the "affected" side. It will be weaker. Use the terms "weaker" or "involved" to refer to the affected side. Never refer to the weaker side as the "bad" side or talk about the "bad" leg or arm.

- Place the weak arm or leg through the garment first, then the strong arm. When undressing, do the opposite.

Oral Care

GUIDELINES: GOOD ORAL CARE

- Oral care, or care of the mouth, teeth, and gums, is performed at least twice each day.

- Oral care should be done after breakfast and after the last meal or snack of the day.

- Oral care includes brushing teeth and gums and tongue, flossing teeth, and caring for dentures.

When you perform or assist with oral care, observe the client's mouth.

ORAL CARE: OBSERVING AND REPORTING

- irritation

- infection

- raised areas

- coated tongue

- ulcers, such as canker sores or small, painful, white sores

- flaky, white spots

- dry and cracked or chapped lips
- loose or decayed teeth
- swollen, bleeding, or whitish gums
- breath that smells bad or fruity

Assisting with oral care

Equipment: soft-bristled toothbrush, toothpaste or powder, glass of water, two towels, moisturizer for lips, basin and a drinking straw (if the client is in bed), gloves

1 Wash your hands.

2 Explain the procedure to the client. Speak clearly, slowly, and directly. Maintain face-to-face contact whenever possible.

3 Provide privacy for the client.

4 If your client is in bed, have him sit up, propped up by pillows. If the bed is adjustable, adjust bed to a safe working level, usually waist high. If bed is movable, lock bed wheels. Place a towel under your client's head and one across the chest.

5 Put on gloves.

6 Remove any dental bridgework or ask your client to do so.

7 Wet toothbrush and put a small amount of toothpaste on it.

8 Gently brush the teeth, or help the client brush teeth. Use short strokes and brush back and forth on all surfaces. Brush the tongue gently as well.

9 Give the client water to rinse the mouth and place the basin under the client's chin for him to spit the water into.

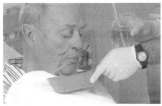

10 Replace any dental bridgework. Apply moisturizer to the lips if the client desires.

11 Put the soiled towels in the laundry hamper. Dispose of the water in the basin by pouring it into the toilet. Clean the basin and put away supplies. Remove your gloves and discard them. If you raised an adjustable bed, return it to its lowest position.

12 Wash your hands.

13 Document the procedure and any observations. Did you observe any mouth ulcers or other broken skin? What was the condition of the mucous membrane? Did the client's breath smell unusual?

Even though unconscious clients cannot eat, breathing through the mouth causes saliva to dry in the mouth. Good oral care needs to be performed more frequently to keep the mouth clean and moist. Swabs with a mixture of lemon juice and glycerine are sometimes used to soothe the gums. However, these may further dry the gums if used too often. Follow the care plan regarding the use of swabs.

With unconscious clients, it is important to use as little liquid as possible when performing oral care. Because the person's swallowing reflex is weak, he or she is at risk for aspiration. Aspiration is the inhalation of food or drink into the lungs. Aspiration can cause pneumonia or death.

Performing oral care for the unconscious client

Equipment: sponge swabs, lemon glycerine swabs (optional), padded tongue blade, mouthwash, emesis basin or small bowl, towel, glass of cool water, lip moisturizer, gloves

1   Wash your hands.

2   Explain the procedure to the client. Speak clearly, slowly, and directly. Maintain face-to-face contact whenever possible. Even clients who are unconscious may be able to hear you. Always speak to them as you would to any client.

3   Provide privacy for the client.

4   If the bed is adjustable, adjust bed to a safe working level, usually waist high. If the bed is movable, lock bed wheels.

5   Put on gloves.

6   Turn your client's head to the side and place a towel under his cheek and chin. Place emesis basin or bowl next to the cheek and chin so that excess fluid flows into the basin.

7   Dip sponge swab in the mouthwash. Do not dip a lemon glycerine swab in mouthwash.

8   Separate the upper and lower teeth with the padded tongue blade. Using the swab, cleanse all surfaces in the mouth cavity,

including the teeth and underneath the tongue. Remove debris with the swab. Rinse and rewet swab as necessary. Repeat this step until the mouth is clean.

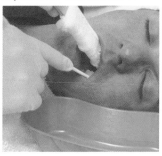

9   If ordered, swab again, this time with the lemon glycerine swab.

10 Remove the towel and basin. Pat lips or face dry if needed. Apply lip moisturizer.

11 Place the towel in the laundry hamper. Clean the basin and put away supplies. Remove your gloves and discard them. If you raised an adjustable bed, return it to its proper position.

12 Wash your hands.

13 Document the procedure and your observations. Did you observe any mouth ulcers or other broken skin? What was the condition of the mucous membrane? Did the client's breath smell unusual?

Flossing the teeth removes plaque and tartar buildup around the gum line and between the teeth. Teeth may be flossed immediately after or before they are brushed. Follow the client's preference.

Flossing teeth

Equipment: about 18 inches of dental floss, glass of water, emesis basin, face towel, gloves

1   Wash your hands.

2   Explain the procedure to the client. Speak clearly, slowly, and directly. Maintain face-to-face contact whenever possible.

3   Provide privacy for the client.

4   Position the client as you would for brushing teeth. If the bed is adjustable, adjust bed to a safe working level, usually waist high. If the bed is movable, lock bed wheels.

5   Put on gloves.

6   Wrap the ends of the floss securely around each of your index fingers.

7   Starting with the back teeth, place the floss between teeth and move it down the surface of the tooth using a gentle sawing motion. Continue to the gum line. At the gum line, curve the floss into a letter C, slip it gently into the space between the gum and tooth, then go back up, scraping that side of the tooth. Repeat this on the side of the other tooth.

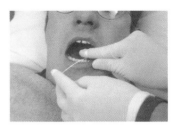

8   After every two or three teeth, unwind floss from your fingers and move it so you are using a clean area. Floss all teeth.

9   Occasionally offer water so that the client can rinse debris from the mouth into the basin.

10 Offer the client a face towel when done flossing all teeth.

11 Discard floss. Pour water from the basin into the toilet. Clean and store the basin. Put the soiled face towel in the laundry hamper. Remove your gloves and discard them. If you raised an adjustable bed, return it to its proper position.

12 Wash your hands.

13 Document procedure and observations.

Remember to ask the client how you can assist with denture care. Each person has his own preference about when and how denture care should be done.

Assisting with denture care

Equipment: denture cup for storage, denture cleaner or toothpaste, denture brush or soft toothbrush, two face towels, basin or sink, gauze squares, mouthwash or a sponge swab, gloves

1   Wash your hands.

2   Explain the procedure to the client. Speak clearly, slowly, and directly. Maintain face-to-face contact whenever possible.

3   Provide privacy for the client.

4   Line the sink or a basin with a face towel and fill with water. The towel and water will prevent the dentures from breaking if they slip from your hands and fall into the sink.

5   Put on gloves.

6   Ask the client to remove the dentures and place them in the denture cup. If the client is unable to remove them, do it yourself. Remove the lower denture first. The lower denture is easier to remove because it floats on the gum line of the lower jaw. Grasp the lower denture with a gauze square (for a good

grip) and remove it. Place it in a denture cup filled with water.

7 The upper denture is sealed by suction. Firmly grasp the upper denture with a gauze square and give a slight downward pull to break the suction. Turn it at an angle to take it out of the mouth.

8 Take the denture cup to the sink or basin. Apply denture cleanser to a denture brush or soft tooth-brush. Brush the dentures under warm, running tap water to remove all material. Do not use hot water, or dentures may warp. Rinse out the denture cup and place dentures in it.

9 Your client may prefer to clean the dentures with a soaking solution. Read the directions on the bottle and prepare the solution. Soak the dentures for the amount of time indicated. Rinse and place in denture cup.

10 Store dentures in water or solution to prevent them from warping. To avoid accidently throwing dentures away, always store them in a labeled denture cup when the client is not wearing them.

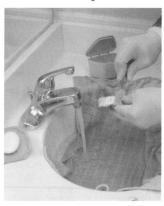

11 Offer the client mouthwash or a swab to cleanse the mouth.

12 Discard gauze pads and swabs. Put towels in laundry hamper. Clean out sink or basin. Rinse and store toothbrush and other supplies. Remove your gloves.

13 Wash your hands.

14 Document procedure and any observations.

Reinserting dentures

Equipment: denture cup with dentures, denture cream or adhesive, face towel, gloves

Ask if the client needs your assistance in inserting dentures.

1 Wash your hands.

2 Explain the procedure to the client. Speak clearly, slowly, and directly. Maintain face-to-face contact whenever possible.

3 Provide privacy for the client.

4 Position client as you would for brushing teeth (help her to as upright a position as possible).

5 Put on gloves.

6 Apply denture cream or adhesive to the dentures if needed.

7 Ask client to open her mouth. Insert the upper denture into the mouth by turning it at an angle. Straighten it and press it onto the upper gum line firmly and evenly.

8 Insert the lower denture onto the gum line of the lower jaw and press firmly.

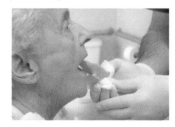

9 Offer the client the face towel.

10 Rinse and store the denture cup. Remove the gloves and discard them.

11 Wash your hands.

12 Document the procedure and any observations.

Toileting

Clients who are unable to get out of bed to go to the bathroom may be given a bedpan, a fracture pan, or a urinal. A fracture pan is a bedpan that is flatter than a regular bedpan. It is used for clients who cannot assist with raising their hips onto a regular bedpan. Men will generally use a urinal for urination and a bedpan for a bowel movement. Rinse this equipment with a disinfectant after each use. Keep the equipment in the bathroom between uses. A spray bottle with a diluted household disinfectant is an easy and sanitary way to keep toileting equipment clean. Hand rails can also be installed next to the toilet. If the client is weak, place a call bell near the toilet.

Remember that wastes such as urine and feces can carry infection. Always dispose of wastes in the toilet. Be careful not to spill or splash. Wear gloves when handling bedpans, urinals, or basins that contain wastes, including dirty bath water. Wash these containers thoroughly with a household disinfectant. After washing these containers, remove your gloves and wash your hands. Put on a new pair of gloves if you are not finished with client care. Commodes should also be cleaned at least once a week.

Washcloths used to wash perineal areas must be washed in hot water. Handle such laundry carefully, and wear gloves. Washing it separately is safest. Disposable washcloths may or may not be flushable. Read the package to be sure. If they are not flushable, dispose of them in a waste container lined with a plastic bag. Remove and replace the plastic bag frequently to prevent odors.

Assisting clients in using a bedpan

Equipment: bedpan, bedpan cover (newspaper or washable cloth), protective pad or sheet, bath blanket, toilet paper, disposable washcloths or wipes, soap, towel, plastic bag, three pairs of gloves

1 Wash your hands.

2 Explain the procedure to the client. Speak clearly, slowly, and directly. Maintain face-to-face contact whenever possible.

3 Provide privacy by closing doors and shades and using a covering blanket.

4 If the bed is adjustable, adjust bed to a safe working level, usually

waist high. If the bed is movable, lock bed wheels. Lower the head of the bed before placing bedpan.

5 Put on gloves.

6 Warm outside of the bedpan with warm water in the bathroom and cover it when you bring it to the client. Dust the top of the bedpan with talcum powder to prevent it from sticking to the client's skin. Do not use talcum powder if the client has open sores on the buttocks or genitals. Do not use powder if a urine or stool sample is needed. If a stool or urine sample is not needed, place a few sheets of toilet paper in the bedpan to make cleanup easier.

7 Cover the client with the bath blanket and ask him to hold it while you pull down the top covers underneath it.

8 Place a protective sheet under the client. To do this, have the client roll toward you. If the client is unable to roll toward you unassisted, you must roll the client. Be sure the client cannot roll off the bed. Move to the empty side of the bed and place the protective sheet on the area where the client will lie on his back. The side of the protective sheet nearest the client should be fanfolded (folded several times into pleats). Ask the client to roll onto his back, or roll him as you did before. Unfold the rest of the protective sheet so it completely covers the area under and around the client's hips.

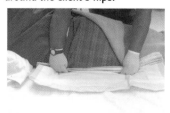

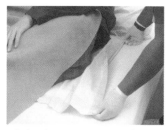

9 Ask the client to remove undergarments, or help him do so.

10 Place the bedpan near his hips with the open end facing the foot of the bed.

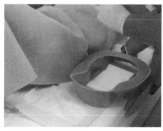

11 Ask the client to help by raising his hips at the count of three. Slide the bedpan under his hips.

If the client cannot do this himself, place your arm under the small of his back and tell him to push with his heels and hands on your signal as you raise his hips. If a client cannot help you in any way, keep the bed flat and roll the client onto the far side. Slip the bedpan under the hips and roll the client back onto the bedpan. Then raise the head of the bed after placing the bedpan under the client. Prop the client into a semi-sitting position using pillows.

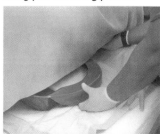

12 Check the bedpan to be certain it is in the correct position. Make sure the bath blanket is still covering the client. Provide the client with toilet paper, washcloths or wipes, and a bell or other way to call you. Tell the client you will return when called. Make sure the client is comfortable before you leave.

13 If the client is unable to clean the anal area and the rest of the perineum, you must do this. With gloves on, help the client to roll onto his side. Use the toilet paper to clean the perineal area first. For female clients, wipe from the front to the back. Use one washcloth to cleanse the front part of the perineum and another to cleanse the anal area.

14 Wrap the toilet paper and disposable washcloths in a plastic bag and discard them. Dry the perineal area with a towel. Place the towel in a hamper. Remove your gloves and discard them. Immediately replace gloves with a clean pair.

15 Offer a wet washcloth and soap and water to the client to wash hands. Cover the client and remove the bath blanket. Help the client put on undergarment.

16 Cover the bedpan and take it to the bathroom. Empty the bedpan carefully into the toilet and flush. If you notice anything unusual about the stool or urine (for example, the presence of blood), do not discard it. Remove and discard your gloves, wash your hands, and notify your supervisor. He or she may ask you to save a specimen. Put on new gloves.

17 Turn the faucet on with a paper towel. Rinse the bedpan with cold water first and empty it into the toilet. Then clean the bedpan with hot, soapy water. Use an approved disinfectant. Store bedpan.

18 Remove and discard gloves. If you raised an adjustable bed, be sure to return it to its proper position.

19 Wash your hands.

20 Document the time of the elimination, the contents, and any observations.

Assisting clients in using a urinal

Equipment: urinal, protective pad or sheet, bath blanket, washcloth, soap, towel, gloves

1 Wash your hands.

2 Explain the procedure to the client. Speak clearly, slowly, and directly. Maintain face-to-face contact whenever possible.

3 Provide privacy by closing doors and shades and using a covering blanket.

4 If the bed is adjustable, adjust bed to a safe working level, usually waist high. If the bed is movable, lock bed wheels.

5 Put on gloves.

6 Place a protective pad under the client's buttocks and hips.

7 Hand the urinal to the client. If the client is not able to help himself, place the urinal between his legs and position the penis inside the urinal. Replace covers.

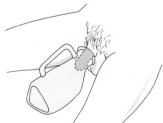

8 Give the client a bell or another way to call you. Leave the room and close the door.

9 When the client signals that he is finished, remove the urinal or

have him hand it to you. Follow the correct procedure if a specimen has been ordered. Discard urine in the toilet. Use a paper towel to turn on the faucet. Rinse the urinal with cold water and use an approved disinfectant. Store it.

10 Remove your gloves and discard them. Wash your hands.

11 Give the client a washcloth, soap, and water to wash his hands.

12 After taking the washcloth from the client and placing it aside (to be washed separately from other laundry), wash your hands again. If you raised an adjustable bed, return it to its proper position.

13 Document the time, the amount of urine (if monitoring intake and output), and any other observations.

Assisting clients in using a portable commode or toilet

Equipment: toilet paper, disposable washcloths or wipes, soap, washcloth, and basin (if using portable commode), gloves

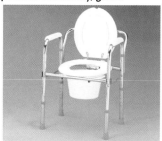

(Photo Courtesy of Nova Ortho Med Inc.)

1 Wash your hands.

2 Explain the procedure to the client. Speak clearly, slowly, and directly. Maintain face-to-face contact whenever possible.

3 Provide privacy by closing doors and shades and using a covering blanket.

4 If the bed is adjustable, adjust bed to a safe working level, usually waist high. If the bed is movable, lock bed wheels.

5 Put on gloves.

6 Help client out of bed and to the bathroom or portable commode.

7 If needed, help client remove clothing and sit on toilet seat.

8 Provide privacy. Leave the room or area. Close the door, but do not lock it. Provide a bell or another way for the client to call you. Do not go too far away in case you are needed soon.

9 When the client calls you, return. If assistance is needed to clean the perineal area, provide it. Remember to wipe female clients from front to back. Use disposable washcloths if necessary. Dispose of these in the toilet, or in the wastebasket if they are not flushable. If your gloves become soiled, discard them and put on fresh gloves.

10 Help the client up and be sure she washes her hands before returning to bed. Use the sink or a basin, soap, and a washcloth.

11 When using a portable commode, remove waste container and empty it into the toilet unless a specimen is needed or the client's urine is being measured for intake/output monitoring. Clean the container as you would a bedpan, rinsing first with cold water and then washing with hot water and cleanser. Use approved disinfectant.

12 Remove your gloves and discard them. If you raised an adjustable bed, return it to its proper position.

13 Wash your hands.

14 Document the procedure and any observations.

13. Vital Signs

You will monitor, document, and report your clients' vital signs. Vital signs are important. They show how well the vital organs of the body, such as the heart and lungs, are working. They consist of the following:

- taking the body temperature

- counting the pulse

- counting the rate of respirations

- taking the blood pressure

- observing and reporting the level of pain

Watching for changes in vital signs is very important. Changes can indicate a client's condition is worsening. Always notify your supervisor if:

- the client is running a fever

- the client has a respiratory or pulse rate that is too rapid or too slow

- the client's blood pressure changes

- the client's pain is worse or is not relieved by pain management

Temperature

Body temperature is normally very close to 98.6°F (Fahrenheit) or 37°C (Celsius). Body temperature reflects a balance between the heat created by our bodies and the heat lost to the environment. Increases in body temperature may indicate an infection or disease. There are four sites for taking body temperature:

1 the mouth (oral)

2 the rectum (rectal)

3 the armpit (axillary)

4 the ear (tympanic)

The different sites require different thermometers. Temperatures are most often taken orally. Remember that there is a range of normal temperatures. Some people's temperatures normally run low. Others in completely good health will run slightly higher temperatures. Normal temperature readings also vary according to the method used to take the temperature.

Normal Ranges for Vital Signs

TEMPERATURE:	FAHRENHEIT	CELSIUS
Oral	97.6°–99.6°	36.5°–37.5°
Rectal	98.6°–100.6°	37.0°–38.1°
Axillary	96.6°–98.6°	36.0°–37.0°

Pulse: 60–90 beats per minute
Respirations: 12–20 respirations per minute
Blood Pressure: Systolic 100–119, Diastolic 60–79 *

* Millions of people whose blood pressure was previously normal (120/80) now fall into the "prehypertension" range. Prehypertension means that the person does not have high blood pressure now but is likely to have it in the future. This is based on the new, more aggressive high blood pressure guidelines from the Seventh Report of the Joint National Committee (JNC 7) on Prevention, Detection, Evaluation, and Treatment of High Blood Pressure (2003).

Types of thermometers are:

- Mercury-free
- Glass bulb (mercury) *
- Oral, rectal, or axillary
- Battery-powered, digital, or electronic
- Tympanic (ear)

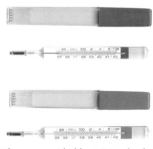

(Photos provided by RG Medical Diagnostics of Southfield, MI.)

* Using glass bulb or mercury thermometers to take oral or rectal temperatures used to be common. However, because mercury is a dangerous, toxic substance, thousands of healthcare facilities now discourage the use of products containing mercury. In fact, many states have passed laws to ban the sale of mercury thermometers.

Mercury-free thermometers are becoming more common. They can be used to take an oral or rectal temperature, and they are considered much safer. Mercury-free thermometers can usually be purchased at your local pharmacy.

Taking and recording an oral temperature

Do not take an oral temperature on a client who has smoked, eaten or drunk fluids, or exercised in the last 10-20 minutes.

Equipment: mercury-free, glass, digital, or electronic thermometer, disposable plastic sheath/cover for thermometer, tissues, pen and paper

1 Wash your hands.

2 Explain the procedure to the client. Speak clearly, slowly, and directly. Maintain face-to-face contact whenever possible.

3 Provide privacy for the client.

Using a mercury-free thermometer or glass thermometer:

4 Hold the thermometer by the stem.

5 Before inserting the thermometer in client's mouth, shake thermometer down to below the lowest number (at least below 96°F or 35°C). To shake the thermometer down, hold it at the side opposite the bulb with the thumb and two fingers. With a snapping motion of the wrist, shake the thermometer. Stand away from furniture and walls while doing so.

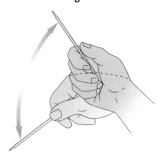

6 Put on disposable sheath, if available. Insert fluted tip or bulb end of the thermometer into client's mouth, under tongue and to one side.

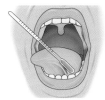

7 Tell the client to hold the thermometer in mouth with lips closed. Assist as necessary. Client should breathe through his or her nose. Ask the client not to bite down or talk.

8 Leave the thermometer in place for at least three minutes.

9 Remove the thermometer. Wipe with a tissue from stem to bulb or remove sheath. Dispose of the tissue or sheath.

10 Hold the thermometer at eye level. Rotate until line appears, rolling the thermometer between your thumb and forefinger. Read the temperature. Document the temperature, date, time and method used (oral).

11 Rinse the thermometer in lukewarm water and dry. Return it to plastic case or container. If using a mercury/glass thermometer, store it away from a heat source.

Using a digital thermometer:

4 Put on the disposable sheath.

5 Turn on thermometer and wait until "ready" sign appears.

6 Insert the end of digital thermometer into client's mouth, under tongue and to one side.

7 Leave in place until thermometer blinks or beeps.

8 Remove the thermometer.

9 Read temperature on display screen. Document the temperature, date, time and method used (oral).

10 Using a tissue, remove and dispose of sheath.

11 Replace the thermometer in case.

Using an electronic thermometer:

4 Remove the probe from base unit.

5 Put on probe cover.

6 Insert the end of electronic thermometer into client's mouth, under tongue and to one side.

7   Leave in place until you hear a tone or see a flashing or steady light.

8   Read the temperature on the display screen.

9   Remove the probe. Press the eject button to discard the cover.

10 Document the temperature, date, time and method used (oral).

11 Return the probe to the holder.

Final step for all thermometers:

12 Wash your hands.

Taking and recording a rectal temperature

You need the client's cooperation to take a rectal temperature. Advise the client to hold still. Reassure him or her that the procedure will only take a few minutes. Hold onto the thermometer at all times while taking a rectal temperature.

Equipment: rectal mercury-free, glass, or digital thermometer, lubricant, gloves, tissue, disposable plastic sheath/cover, pen and paper

1   Wash your hands.

2   Explain the procedure to the client. Speak clearly, slowly, and directly. Maintain face-to-face contact whenever possible.

3   Provide privacy for the client.

4   Assist the client to a side-lying position, with his back to you and knees slightly bent. An infant can be placed on his back or stomach for measuring rectal temperature.

5   Fold back the linens to expose only the rectal area.

6   Put on gloves.

7   *Mercury-free or glass thermometer:* Hold thermometer by stem.

    Digital thermometer: Apply probe cover.

8   *Mercury-free or glass thermometer:* Shake the thermometer down to below the lowest number.

9   Apply a small amount of lubricant to tip or bulb or probe cover.

10 Separate the buttocks. Gently insert thermometer into rectum 1 inch (1/2 inch for a child). Stop if

you meet resistance. Do not force the thermometer in.

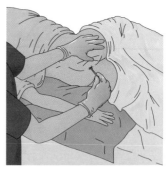

11 Replace the sheet over buttocks while holding onto the thermometer. Hold onto the thermometer at all times while taking a rectal temperature.

12 *Mercury-free or glass thermometer:* Hold thermometer in place for at least three minutes.

    Digital thermometer: Hold thermometer in place until thermometer blinks or beeps.

13 Gently remove the thermometer. Wipe with tissue from stem to bulb or remove sheath. Dispose of tissue or sheath.

14 Read the thermometer at eye level as you would for an oral temperature. Document the temperature, date, time and method used (rectal).

15 *Mercury-free or glass thermometer:* Rinse the thermometer in lukewarm water and dry. Return it to plastic case or container. If using a mercury/glass thermometer, store it away from a heat source.

Digital thermometer: Throw away probe cover and return thermometer to storage area.

16 Remove and dispose of gloves.

17 Assist the client to a position of safety and comfort.

18 Wash your hands.

Taking and recording a tympanic temperature

Equipment: tympanic thermometer, disposable probe sheath/cover, pen and paper

1 Wash your hands.

2 Explain procedure to client, speaking clearly, slowly, and directly, maintaining face-to-face contact whenever possible.

3 Provide privacy for the client.

4 Put a disposable sheath over earpiece of the thermometer.

5 Position the client's head so that the ear is in front of you. Straighten the ear canal by pulling up and back on the outside edge of the ear for an adult. Pull straight back for infants and children. Insert the covered probe into the ear canal and press the button.

6 Hold thermometer in place either

for one second or until thermometer beeps (depends on model).

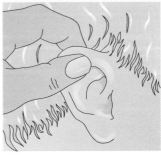

7 Read temperature. Document the temperature, date, time and method used (tympanic).

8 Dispose of sheath. Return the thermometer to storage or to the battery charger if thermometer is rechargeable.

9 Wash your hands.

Taking and recording an axillary temperature

Axillary temperatures are much less reliable than temperatures taken at other sites. The axillary site is usually used as a last resort.

Equipment: mercury-free, glass, digital, or electronic thermometer, tissues, disposable sheath/cover, pen and paper

1 Wash your hands.

2 Explain the procedure to the client. Speak clearly, slowly, and directly. Maintain face-to-face contact whenever possible.

3 Provide privacy for the client.

4 Remove the client's arm from sleeve of gown. Wipe axillary area with tissues.

Using a mercury-free thermometer or glass thermometer:

5 Hold thermometer at stem end. Shake down to below the lowest number.

6 Put the disposable sheath on thermometer, if applicable.

7 Place bulb end of thermometer in center of armpit. Fold the client's arm over chest.

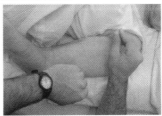

8   Hold in place, with the arm close against the side, for 10 minutes.

9   Remove the thermometer. Wipe with tissue from stem to bulb or remove sheath. Dispose of tissue or sheath.

10 Hold thermometer at eye level. Rotate until line appears and read temperature. Record temperature, date, time, and method used (axillary).

11 Clean thermometer and/or return it to container for used thermometers.

Using a digital thermometer:

5   Put on disposable sheath. Turn on thermometer. Wait until "ready" sign appears.

6   Position end of digital thermometer in center of armpit. Fold the client's arm over chest.

7   Hold in place until thermometer blinks or beeps.

8   Remove the thermometer.

9   Read temperature on display screen. Record the temperature, date, time, and method used (axillary).

10 Using a tissue, remove and dispose of sheath.

11 Replace thermometer in case.

Using an electronic thermometer:

5   Remove probe from base unit. Put on probe cover.

6   Position end of electronic thermometer in center of armpit. Fold the client's arm over chest.

7   Leave in place until you hear a tone or see a flashing or steady light.

8   Read the temperature on the display screen.

9   Remove the probe. Press the eject button to discard the cover.

10 Record temperature, date, time, and method used (axillary).

11 Return the probe to the holder.

Final steps:

12 Put the client's arm back into sleeve and make him or her comfortable.

13 Wash your hands.

Pulse

The pulse is essentially the number of heartbeats per minute. The beat that you feel at certain pulse points in the body represents the wave of blood moving as a result of the heart pumping. The most common site for monitoring the pulse is on the inside of the wrist, where the radial artery runs just beneath the skin. This is called the radial pulse.

For adults, the normal pulse rate is 60-90 beats per minute. Small children have more rapid pulses, in the range of 100-120 beats per minute. A newborn baby's pulse may be as high as 120-140 beats per minute. Many things can affect the pulse rate, including exercise, fear, anger, anxiety, heat, medications, and pain. An unusually high or low rate does not necessarily indicate disease. However, sometimes the pulse rate can be a signal that serious illness exists. For example, a rapid pulse may result from fever, infection, or heart failure. A slow or weak pulse may indicate dehydration, infection, or shock.

The apical (AY-pi-kul) pulse is heard by listening directly over the heart with a stethoscope. This is often the easiest method for measuring the pulse in infants and small children because their pulse points are harder to find. A stethoscope is an instrument designed to listen to sounds within the body, such as the heart beating or air moving through the lungs.

Taking and recording apical pulse

Equipment: stethoscope, watch with second hand

1 Wash your hands.

2 Explain the procedure to the client. Speak clearly, slowly, and directly. Maintain face-to-face contact whenever possible.

3 Provide privacy for the client.

4 Fit the earpieces of the stethoscope snugly in your ears. Place the flat metal diaphragm on the left side of the chest, just below the nipple. Listen for the heartbeat.

5 Use the second hand of your watch. Count the heartbeats for one minute. Each "lubdub" that you hear is counted as one beat. A

normal heartbeat is rhythmical. Leave the stethoscope in place to count respirations (see procedure later in chapter).

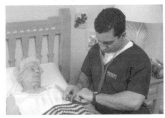

6 Document the pulse rate, date, time, and method used (apical). Note any irregularities in the rhythm.

7 Store stethoscope.

8 Wash your hands.

Respirations

Respiration is the process of breathing air into the lungs, or inspiration, and exhaling air out of the lungs, or expiration. Each respiration consists of an inspiration and an expiration. The chest rises during inspiration and falls during expiration.

The normal respiration rate for adults ranges from 12 to 20 breaths per minute. Infants and children have a faster respiratory rate; infants can breathe normally at a rate of 30-40 respirations per minute. People may breathe more quickly if they know they are being observed. Because of this, count respirations immediately after taking the pulse. Keep your fingers on the client's wrist or on the stethoscope over the heart. Do not make it obvious that you are observing the client's breathing.

Taking and recording radial pulse, and counting and recording respirations

Equipment: watch with a second hand

1 Wash your hands.

2 Explain the procedure to the client. Speak clearly, slowly, and directly. Maintain face-to-face contact whenever possible.

3 Provide privacy for the client.

4 Place fingertips on the thumb side of client's wrist to locate pulse.

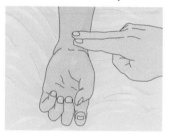

5 Count the beats for one full minute.

6 Keeping your fingertips on the client's wrist, count respirations for one full minute. Observe for the pattern and character of the client's breathing. Normal breathing is smooth and quiet. If you see signs of difficult breathing, shallow breathing, or noisy breathing, such as wheezing, report it to your supervisor.

7 Document the pulse rate, date, time, and method used (radial). Notify your supervisor if the pulse is less than 60 beats per minute, over 90 beats per minute, or if the rhythm is irregular. Document the respiratory rate and the pattern or character of breathing.

8 Wash your hands.

Blood Pressure

Blood pressure is an important indicator of a person's health. Blood pressure is measured in millimeters of mercury (mmHg). The measurement shows how well the heart is working. There are two parts of blood pressure, the systolic (sis-TOL-ik) and diastolic (DYE-a-stol-ik).

In the systolic phase, the heart is at work, contracting and pushing the blood from the left ventricle of the heart. The reading you get shows the pressure on the walls of arteries as blood is pumped through the body. The normal range for systolic blood pressure is 100 to 119 mmHg.

The second measurement reflects the diastolic phase—when the heart relaxes. The diastolic measurement is always lower than the systolic measurement. It shows the pressure in the arteries when the heart is at rest. The normal range for adults is 60 to 79 mmHg.

People with high blood pressure, or hypertension, have elevated systolic and/or diastolic blood pressures. A blood pressure level of 140/90 mmHg or higher is considered high.

However, if blood pressure is between 120/80 mmHg and 139/89 mmHg, it is called prehypertension. This person does not have high blood pressure now but is likely to have it in the future. Report to your supervisor if a client's blood pressure is 140/90 or above.

Taking blood pressure (two-step method)

Equipment: sphygmomanometer (blood pressure cuff), stethoscope, alcohol wipes, pen and paper

1 Wash your hands.

2 Explain the procedure to the client. Speak clearly, slowly, and directly. Maintain face-to-face contact whenever possible.

3 Provide privacy for the client.

4 Ask the client to roll up his or her sleeve. Do not measure blood pressure over clothing.

5 Position the client's arm with the palm up. The arm should be level with the heart.

6 With the valve open, squeeze the cuff to make sure it is completely deflated.

7 Place the blood pressure cuff snugly on client's upper arm, with the center of the cuff placed over the brachial artery (1-1½ inches above the elbow toward inside of elbow).

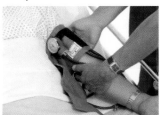

8 Locate the radial (wrist) pulse with your fingertips.

9 Close the valve (clockwise) until it stops. Inflate the cuff while watching the gauge.

10 Stop inflating when you can no longer feel the radial pulse. Note the reading. The number is an estimate of the systolic pressure. This estimate helps you not to inflate the cuff too high later in this procedure. Inflating the cuff too high is painful and may damage small blood vessels.

11 Open the valve to deflate cuff completely. An inflated cuff left on client's arm can cause numbness and tingling.

12 Write down the systolic reading.

13 Before using the stethoscope, wipe the diaphragm and earpieces of stethoscope with alcohol wipes.

14 Locate the brachial pulse with fingertips.

15 Place the earpieces of the stethoscope in your ears.

16 Place the diaphragm of the stethoscope over the brachial artery.

17 Close the valve (clockwise) until it stops. Do not tighten it.

18 Inflate the cuff to 30 mmHg above your estimated systolic pressure.

19 Open the valve slightly with thumb and index finger. Deflate cuff slowly. Releasing the valve slowly allows you to hear beats accurately.

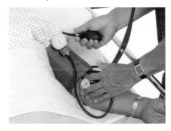

20 Watch the gauge and listen for sound of pulse.

21 Remember the reading at which

the first clear pulse sound is heard. This is the systolic pressure.

22 Continue listening for a change or muffling of pulse sound. The point of a change or the point at which the sound disappears is the diastolic pressure. Remember this reading.

23 Open the valve to deflate cuff completely. Remove cuff.

24 Document both systolic and diastolic pressures. Write the numbers like a fraction, with the systolic reading on top and the diastolic reading on the bottom (for example: 120/80). Note which arm was used. Write "RA" for right arm and "LA" for left arm.

25 Wipe diaphragm and earpieces of stethoscope with alcohol. Store equipment.

26 Wash your hands.

Pain

It is important to observe and report on a client's pain. You play an important role in pain monitoring and prevention. If a client complains of pain, ask these questions to get the most accurate information. Report the information to your supervisor immediately.

• Where is the pain?

• When did the pain start?

• Is the pain mild, moderate or severe? To help assess this, ask the client to rate the pain on a scale of 1 to 10. Ten is the most severe.

• Ask the client to describe the pain. Make notes if you need to and use the client's words when reporting to your supervisor.

• Ask the client what he or she was doing before the pain started.

Measures to reduce pain include the following:

• Report complaints of pain or unrelieved pain promptly to your supervisor.

• Gently position the body in good alignment. Use pillows for support. Assist in frequent changes of position if the client desires it.

• Give back rubs.

• Offer warm baths or showers.

• Assist the client to the bathroom or commode or offer the bedpan or urinal.

• Encourage slow, deep breaths when the client has difficulty breathing.

• Provide a calm and quiet environment. Use soft music to distract the client.

- If a client is taking pain medication, remind him or her when it is time to take it.

- Be patient, caring, gentle, and sympathetic.

You may be asked to check your clients' weight and height as part of your care. Height is checked less frequently than weight. Weight changes can be indicators of illness. You must report any weight loss or gain, no matter how small.

Measuring and recording the weight of a client

Equipment: bathroom scale

1 Wash your hands.

2 Explain the procedure to the client. Speak clearly, slowly, and directly. Maintain face-to-face contact whenever possible.

3 Provide privacy for the client.

4 Set the scale on a hard surface in a place the client can get to easily.

5 Start with the scale balanced at zero before weighing the client. If it does not read zero, adjust the knob.

6 Help client to the scale as needed.

7 Have the client step on the scale.

Assist as needed. Be sure she is not holding, touching, or leaning against anything. This interferes with weight measurement. Do not force someone to let go. If you are unable to obtain a weight, notify your supervisor.

8 When the dial has stopped moving, read the weight.

9 Have the client step off the scale and help her back into a comfortable position.

10 Document the weight.

11 Store the scale if it was moved.

12 Wash your hands.

Measuring and recording the height of a client

Some clients will be unable to get out of bed. For these clients, height can be measured using a tape measure.

Equipment: tape measure and pencil

1 Wash your hands.

2 Explain the procedure to the client. Speak clearly, slowly, and directly. Maintain face-to-face contact whenever possible.

3 Provide privacy for the client.

4 Position the client lying straight in bed, flat on his back with arms and legs at his sides. Be sure the bed sheet is smooth underneath the client.

5 Make a pencil mark on the sheet at the top of the head.

6 Make another mark at the client's heel.

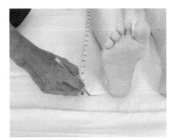

7 With the tape measure, measure the distance between the marks.

8 Document the height.

9   Store equipment.

10 Wash your hands.

For clients who can get out of bed, you will measure height while they stand against a wall.

Equipment: tape measure and pencil

1   Wash your hands.

2   Explain the procedure to the client. Speak clearly, slowly, and directly. Maintain face-to-face contact whenever possible.

3   Provide privacy for the client.

4   Have the client stand with his back to the wall, with his arms at his sides and without shoes. A hard floor is better than carpet.

5   Make a pencil mark on the wall at the top of the client's head.

6   Ask client to step away. Measure the distance between the pencil mark and the floor.

7   Document the height.

8   Store equipment.

9   Wash your hands.

14. Special Procedures

Intake and Output (I&O)

Fluid balance is maintaining intake and output, or taking in and eliminating equal amounts of fluid. Some clients must have their intake and output, or I&O, monitored and documented. To document intake and output, some agencies use a special form called an Intake/Output (I&O) sheet.

Conversions

A cubic centimeter (cc) is a unit of measure that is equal to one milliliter (ml.)

1 oz.	=	30 cc or 30 ml.		
2 oz.	=	60 cc		
3 oz.	=	90 cc		
4 oz.	=	120 cc		
5 oz.	=	150 cc		
6 oz.	=	180 cc		
7 oz.	=	210 cc		
8 oz.	=	240 cc		
1/4 cup	=	2 oz.	=	60 cc
1/2 cup	=	4 oz.	=	120 cc
1 cup	=	8 oz.	=	240 cc

Measuring and recording intake and output

Monitoring fluid balance begins with measuring intake.

Equipment: I&O sheet, graduate (measuring container), pen and paper

1   Wash your hands.

2   Explain the procedure to the client. Speak clearly, slowly, and directly. Maintain face-to-face contact whenever possible.

3   Provide privacy for the client.

4   Using a measuring cup, measure the amount of fluid a client is served. Note the amount on paper, not in the visit notes.

5   When client has finished a meal or snack, measure any leftover fluids. Note this amount on paper.

6   Subtract the leftover amount from the amount served. If you have measured in ounces, convert to cubic centimeters (cc) by multiplying by 30.

7   Document the amount of fluid consumed (in cc) in the visit notes and/or I&O record, as well as the time and what fluid was taken.

Measuring output is the other half of monitoring fluid balance.

Equipment: I&O record, pen and paper, graduate, bedpan, urinal or toilet attachment, plastic bag for disposal of toilet paper, washcloth or towel, gloves

1   Wash your hands.

2   Explain the procedure to the client. Speak clearly, slowly, and directly. Maintain face-to-face contact whenever possible.

3   Provide privacy for the client.

4   Put on gloves.

5   Ask the client to put used toilet paper in the bag, not in the bedpan or toilet. Ask client not to move bowels at the same time as urinating, if possible.

6   Make client comfortable, assisting as necessary. Leave the room if your assistance is not needed.

7   Help the client wash his or her hands using the washcloth and towel.

8   Pour urine into measuring container. Note the amount on paper, converting to cc if necessary.

9   Discard urine. Wash and store equipment. Flush toilet paper down the toilet and discard plastic bag.

10 Remove gloves.

11 Wash your hands.

12 Document the time and amount of urine in output column on sheet. For example: 3:45pm 200 cc urine

Intake & Output Record

Client Name: _____ HHA Name: _____
Address: _____ Record Date: _____

Intake			Output		
Time	Type	Amount	Time	Urine Amount	Incontinent Episode

Output	Time	Approximate Amount
Vomiting		
Heavy Perspiration		
Diarrhea		

Note: To measure vomitus, pour from basin into measuring container, then discard in the toilet. If client vomits on the bed or floor, estimate the amount. Document emesis (EM-e-sis, or vomiting) and amount in the visit notes and/or I&O sheet.

Catheter Care

A catheter is a tube used to drain urine from the bladder. A straight catheter does not remain inside the person. It is removed immediately after urine is drained. An indwelling catheter remains inside the bladder for a period of time. The urine drains into a bag. An external, or condom, catheter has an attachment on the end that fits onto the penis. The external catheter is changed daily.

GUIDELINES: WORKING WITH CLIENTS WHO HAVE CATHETERS

- The drainage bag must always be kept lower than the hips or bladder.

- Tubing should be kept as straight as possible and should not be kinked.

- The genital area must be kept clean to prevent infection. Daily care of the genital area is especially important.

CATHETER CARE: OBSERVING AND REPORTING

- blood in the urine or any other unusual appearance

- catheter bag does not fill after several hours

- catheter bag fills suddenly

- catheter is not in place

- urine leaks from the catheter

- client reports pain

- odor

Providing catheter care

Many clients can clean the catheter site themselves. If you need to provide this care for a client, follow the steps below.

Equipment: bath blanket, protective pad, bath basin, bath thermometer, soap, 2-4 washcloths, 1 towel, gloves

1   Wash your hands.

2   Explain the procedure to the client. Speak clearly, slowly, and directly. Maintain face-to-face contact whenever possible.

3   Provide privacy for the client.

4   If the bed is adjustable, adjust bed to a safe working level, usually waist high.

5   Lower head of bed. Position client lying flat on her back. Raise the side rail farthest from you.

6   Remove or fold back top bedding, keeping client covered with bath blanket.

7   Test water temperature with thermometer or your wrist and ensure it is safe. Water temperature should be 105° to 109°F. Have client check water temperature. Adjust if necessary.

8   Put on gloves.

9   Ask the client to flex her knees and raise the buttocks off the bed by pushing against the mattress with her feet. Place clean protective pad under her buttocks.

10 Expose only the area necessary to clean the catheter.

11 Place towel or pad under catheter tubing before washing.

12 Apply soap to wet washcloth.

13 Hold catheter near meatus to avoid tugging the catheter.

14 Clean at least four inches of catheter nearest meatus. Move in only one direction, away from meatus. Use a clean area of the cloth for each stroke.

15 Dip a clean washcloth in the water. Rinse at least four inches of catheter nearest meatus. Move in only one direction, away from meatus. Use a clean area of the cloth for each stroke.

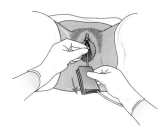

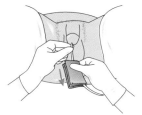

16 Empty the water into the toilet. Dispose of washcloth and towel in proper containers.

17 Remove and dispose of gloves.

18 If you raised an adjustable bed, be sure to return it to its lowest position.

19 Wash your hands.

20 Help the client dress. Arrange covers. Check that the catheter tubing is free from kinks and twists and that it is securely taped to the leg.

21 Wash your hands again.

22 Document procedure and any observations.

Emptying the catheter drainage bag

Equipment: graduate (measuring container), alcohol wipes, paper towels, gloves

1 Wash your hands.

2 Explain the procedure to the client. Speak clearly, slowly, and directly. Maintain face-to-face contact whenever possible.

3 Put on gloves.

4 Place paper towel on the floor under the drainage bag. Place measuring container on the paper towel.

5 Open the drain or spout on the bag so that urine flows out of the bag into the measuring container.

6 When urine has drained, close

spout. Using alcohol wipe, clean the drain spout. Replace the drain in its holder on the bag.

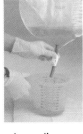

7 Mentally note the amount and the appearance of the urine. Empty into toilet.

8 Clean and store measuring container.

9 Remove gloves.

10 Wash your hands.

11 Document procedure and amount of urine.

Emesis, or vomiting, must be documented. It may be a sign of illness or of a reaction to medication. Some clients, such as those with cancer undergoing chemotherapy, may vomit frequently as a result of treatment. Vomiting is unpleasant. Handle it calmly. Provide comfort to the client.

Observing, reporting, and documenting a client's emesis

Because you may not know when a client is going to vomit, you may not have time to explain what you will do and assemble supplies ahead of time. Talk to the client soothingly as you help him clean up. Tell him what you are doing to help him.

1   Put on gloves when client has vomited.

2   Provide a basin and remove it when vomiting has stopped.

3   Remove soiled linens or clothes. Set aside for laundering. Replace with fresh linens or clothes.

4   If client's I&O is being monitored, measure and note amount of vomitus.

5   Flush vomit down the toilet. Wash and store basin.

6   Remove gloves.

7   Wash your hands.

8   Put on fresh gloves.

9   Provide comfort to client: wipe face and mouth, position comfort-

ably, offer a drink of water or oral care.

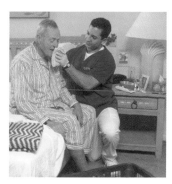

10 Launder soiled linens and clothes promptly in hot water.

11 Remove gloves.

12 Wash your hands again.

13 Document time, amount, color, and consistency of vomitus. Look for blood in vomitus or blood-tinged vomitus.

14 Report to your supervisor immediately and get instructions for diet.

Ostomy Care

An ostomy is a surgical procedure that creates an opening in the body for the discharge of body wastes. In a client with an ostomy, the end of the intestine is brought out of the body through an artificial opening in the abdomen. This opening is called a stoma. Stool, or feces, are eliminated through the ostomy rather than through the anus. The terms colostomy (koh-LOS-toh-mee) and ileostomy (il-ee-OS-toh-mee) indicate what part of the intestine was removed and the type of stool that will be eliminated. In a colostomy, stool will generally be semi-solid. With an ileostomy, stool may be liquid and irritating to the client's skin.

Clients who have had an ostomy wear a disposable bag that fits over the stoma to collect the feces. The bag is attached to the skin by adhesive. Many people manage the ostomy appliance by themselves. Your employer should provide training before you provide this care. If you are providing ostomy care, make certain the client receives good skin care and hygiene. The ostomy bag should be emptied and cleaned or replaced whenever a stool is eliminated. Always wear gloves and wash hands carefully when providing ostomy care. Teach proper handwashing techniques to clients with ostomies.

Caring for an ostomy

Equipment: bedpan, disposable bed protector, bath blanket, clean ostomy bag and belt/appliance, toilet paper, basin of warm water, soap or cleanser, washcloth, skin cream as ordered, two towels, plastic disposable bag, 3 pairs of gloves

1   Wash your hands.

2   Explain the procedure to the client. Speak clearly, slowly, and directly. Maintain face-to-face contact whenever possible.

3   Provide privacy for the client.

4   If the bed is adjustable, adjust bed to a safe working level, usually waist high.

5   Place bed protector under client. Cover client with a bath blanket. Pull down the top sheet and blankets. Only expose the ostomy site. Offer client a towel to keep clothing dry.

6   Put on gloves.

7   Remove ostomy bag carefully. If it will be washed and reused, place it in the bedpan. If it will be discarded, place it in the plastic bag. Note the color, odor, consistency, and amount of stool in the bag.

8   Wipe the area around the stoma with toilet paper. Discard paper in plastic bag.

9   Using a washcloth and warm soapy water, wash the area around the stoma. Pat dry with another

towel. Apply cream as ordered.

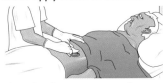

10   Place the clean ostomy appliance on client, following your supervisor's instructions. Make sure the bottom of the bag is clamped.

11   Remove disposable bed protector and discard.

12   Remove gloves. Make the client comfortable. Put on fresh gloves and change linens if necessary. Cover the client and remove bath blanket and towel. Place soiled linens in appropriate containers. Remove gloves.

13   Put on new gloves. Take bedpan and other supplies to bathroom. Empty bag into toilet and flush, along with used toilet paper. Wash out bag. Use a deodorant in the bag as directed.

14   Clean bedpan, pouring rinse water into toilet. Return to proper storage.

15   Remove and dispose of gloves properly.

16   Return bed to appropriate level if previously adjusted.

17   Wash your hands.

18   Document procedure and any observations.

Note: Call your supervisor if stoma appears very red or blue, or if swelling or bleeding is present.

Many clients with ostomies feel they have lost control of a basic bodily function. They may be embarrassed or angry about the ostomy. Be sensitive and supportive when working with these clients. Always provide privacy for ostomy care.

Collecting Specimens

Sometimes you may be asked to collect a specimen from a client. A specimen is a sample of a body secretion. You may be asked to collect these different types of specimens:

- Sputum (SPYOO-tum) is mucus coughed up from the lungs.

- Stool (feces) specimens are another type of sample collected.

- Urine specimens may be routine, clean catch (mid-stream) or 24-hour.

Collecting a sputum specimen

Equipment: specimen container with cover (labeled with client's name, address, date and time), tissues, plastic bag, gloves, mask

1 Wash your hands.

2 Explain the procedure to the client. Speak clearly, slowly, and directly. Maintain face-to-face contact whenever possible.

3 Provide privacy for the client.

4 Put on mask and gloves. If the client has known or suspected tuberculosis or another infectious disease, you should wear a mask when collecting a sputum specimen. Coughing is one way TB germs can enter the air.

5 Ask the client to cough deeply, so that sputum comes up from the lungs. To prevent the spread of infectious material, give the client tissues to cover his or her mouth while coughing. Ask the client to spit the sputum into the specimen container.

6 When you have obtained a good sample (about two tablespoons of sputum), cover the container tightly. Wipe any sputum off the outside of the container with tissues. Discard the tissues. Put the specimen container in the plastic bag and seal.

7 Remove gloves and mask.

8 Wash your hands.

9 Document the procedure.

Collecting a stool specimen

Ask the client to let you know when he or she can have a bowel movement. Be ready to collect the specimen.

Equipment: specimen container and lid with label, 2 tongue blades, 2 pairs of gloves, bedpan, portable commode or toilet attachment (hat), 2 plastic bags, toilet tissue, washcloth or towel, supplies for perineal care

1   Wash your hands.

2   Explain the procedure to the client. Speak clearly, slowly, and directly. Maintain face-to-face contact whenever possible.

3   Provide privacy for the client.

4   Put on gloves.

5   When the client is ready to move bowels, ask him not to urinate at the same time and not to put toilet paper in with the sample. Provide a plastic bag to discard toilet paper separately.

6   Fit hat to toilet or commode, or provide client with bedpan. Leave the room and ask the client to call you when he is finished with the bowel movement.

7   After the bowel movement, assist as necessary with perineal care. Help client wash his or her hands

at the sink or using the washcloth and towel. Make the client comfortable. Remove gloves.

8   Wash your hands again.

9   Put on clean gloves.

10 Using the two tongue blades, take about two tablespoons of stool and put it in the container. Without touching the inside of the container, cover it tightly.

11 Wrap the tongue blades in toilet paper and throw them away. Empty the bedpan or container into the toilet. Clean and store the equipment.

12 Store the specimen properly. It must be bagged and labeled.

13 Remove and dispose of gloves.

14 Wash your hands.

15 Document the procedure. Note amount and characteristics of stool.

Collecting a routine urine specimen

Equipment: urine specimen container and lid, label, gloves, bedpan or urinal (if client cannot use the bathroom), "hat" for toilet (if client can get to the bathroom), 2 plastic bags, washcloth, towel, paper towel, supplies for perineal care, PPE (if needed)

1   Wash your hands.

2   Explain the procedure to the client. Speak clearly, slowly, and directly. Maintain face-to-face contact whenever possible.

3   Provide privacy for the client.

4   Put on gloves.

5   Assist the client to the bathroom or commode, or offer the bedpan or urinal.

6   Have client void into "hat," urinal, or bedpan. Ask the client not to put toilet paper in with the sample. Provide a plastic bag to discard toilet paper separately.

7   After urination, assist as necessary with perineal care. Help client wash his or her hands at the sink or using the washcloth and towel. Make the client comfortable.

8   Take bedpan, urinal, or commode pail to the bathroom.

9   Pour urine from bedpan, urinal, or toilet attachment into the specimen container. Specimen container should be at least half full.

10 Cover the urine container with its lid. Wipe off the outside with a paper towel.

11 Place the container in a plastic bag.

12 If using a bedpan or urinal, discard extra urine. Rinse and clean equipment, and store.

13 Remove and dispose of gloves.

14 Complete the label for the container with the client's name, address, the date, and time.

15 Wash your hands.

16 Document the procedure. Note amount and characteristics of urine.

Some clients will be able to collect their own specimens. Others will need your help. Be sure to explain exactly how the specimen must be collected.

Collecting a clean catch (mid-stream) urine specimen

Equipment: specimen kit with container, label, cleansing solution, gauze or towelettes, gloves, bedpan or urinal (if client cannot use the bathroom), plastic bag, washcloth, paper towel, towel, supplies for perineal care, PPE (if needed)

1 Wash your hands.

2 Explain the procedure to the client. Speak clearly, slowly, and directly. Maintain face-to-face contact whenever possible.

3 Provide privacy for the client.

4 Put on gloves.

5 Open the specimen kit. Do not touch the inside of the container or the inside of the lid.

6 Using the towelettes or gauze and cleansing solution, clean the area around the urethra. *For females*, separate the labia and wipe from front to back along one side. Discard towelette/gauze. With a new towelette or gauze, wipe from front to back along the other labia. Using a new towelette or gauze, wipe down the middle.

For males, clean the head of the penis using circular motions with the towelettes or gauze. Clean thoroughly, changing towelettes/gauze after each circular motion and discarding after use. If the man is uncircumcised,

pull back the foreskin of the penis before cleaning and hold it back during urination. Make sure it is pulled back down after collecting the specimen.

7 Ask the client to urinate into the bedpan, urinal, or toilet, and to stop before urination is complete.

8 Place the container under the urine stream and have the client start urinating again. Fill the container at least half full. Have the client finish urinating in bedpan, urinal, or toilet.

9 Cover the urine container with its lid. Wipe off the outside with a paper towel.

10 Place the container in a plastic bag.

11 If using a bedpan or urinal, discard extra urine. Rinse and clean equipment, and store.

12 After urination, assist as necessary with perineal care. Remove and dispose of gloves. Wash your hands. Help client wash his hands at the sink or using the washcloth.

13 Complete the label for the container with the client's name and address, the date, and time.

14 Wash your hands again.

15 Document the procedure. Note amount and characteristics of urine.

Collecting a 24-hour urine specimen

Since you will probably not be present during all 24 hours of the test, it is important to explain the

collection fully to the client and family members.

Equipment: container for urine (gallon bottle or a container from the lab), bedpan or urinal (for clients confined to bed), "hat" for toilet (if client can get to the bathroom), bucket of ice (if the urine must be kept cold) or a clearly-marked container can also be put in the refrigerator, funnel (if the container opening is small), gloves, washcloth or towel, supplies for perineal care, PPE (if needed)

1 Wash your hands.

2 Explain the procedure to the client. Speak clearly, slowly, and directly. Maintain face-to-face contact whenever possible.

3 Provide privacy for the client.

4 When beginning the collection, have the client completely empty the bladder. Discard the urine and note the exact time of this voiding. The collection will run until the same time tomorrow.

5 Label the container with client's name, address, dates and times the collection period began and ended.

6 Put on gloves each time the client voids.

7 Pour urine from bedpan, urinal, or toilet attachment into the container, using the funnel as needed.

8 After each voiding, assist as necessary with perineal care. Help the client wash his or her hands using the washcloth and towel after each voiding.

9 Be sure the client or a family member understands that all urine is to be saved, even when you are gone. Show them how to pour the urine into the container. Remind them to store the container in the bucket of ice or in the refrigerator if ordered.

10 Clean equipment after each voiding.

11 Remove gloves.

12 Wash your hands.

13 Document the time of the last void before the 24-hour collection period began, and the last void of the 24-hour collection period.

Non-Sterile Dressings

Sterile dressings are those that cover open or draining wounds. A nurse changes these dressings. Non-sterile dressings are applied to dry wounds that have less chance of infection. Home health aides may assist with non-sterile dressing changes.

Changing a dry dressing using non-sterile technique

Equipment: package of square gauze dressings, adhesive tape, scissors, 2 pairs of gloves, waste bag

1 Wash your hands.

2 Explain the procedure to the client. Speak clearly, slowly, and directly. Maintain face-to-face contact whenever possible.

3 Provide privacy for the client.

4 Cut pieces of tape long enough to secure the dressing. Hang tape on the edge of a table within reach. Open the four-inch gauze square package without touching the gauze. Place the opened package on a flat surface.

5 Put on gloves.

6   Remove soiled dressing by gently peeling tape toward the wound. Lift dressing off the wound. Do not drag it over the wound. Observe the dressing for odor or drainage. Notice the color of the wound. Dispose of used dressing in the waste bag. Remove your gloves. Place them in the waste bag.

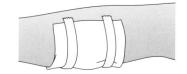

7   Put on new gloves. Touching only outer edges of new four-inch gauze, remove it from package. Apply it to the wound. Tape gauze in place. Secure it firmly.

8   Remove gloves. Discard in the waste bag.

9   Wash your hands.

10   Document the procedure and your observations.

Heat and Cold Applications

Applying heat or cold to injured areas can have several good effects. Heat tends to relieve pain and muscular tension. It reduces swelling, elevates the temperature in the tissues, and increases blood flow. Increased blood flow brings more oxygen and nutrients to the tissues for healing.

Cold applications can help stop bleeding. They prevent swelling, reduce pain, and bring down high fevers.

Never perform a procedure you are not trained to do. Only perform procedures that are assigned to you.

Be alert for excessive redness, pain, blisters, or numbness at the site of a heat or cold application. If you observe these signs, the application may be causing tissue damage. Report any of these signs to your supervisor.

Electric heating pads can also be used as heat applications. Follow the care plan. Do not use a heating pad unless it has been ordered in the care plan or by your supervisor.

GUIDELINES: USING A HEATING PAD

- Check the skin frequently for redness or pain. Electric heating pads do not cool down. Having it just a little too hot can be very dangerous for the client.

- Make sure any electric heating pad you use is in good shape. Do not use it if the cord is frayed or if wires are exposed.

- Do not use a pin to fasten the pad. The pin could contact a wire inside the pad and cause a shock.

- Do not allow the client to lie on top of an electric heating pad.

- Do not allow the client to use an electric heating pad near a source of water.

Another type of heat application is a sitz bath, or a warm soak of the perineal area. Sitz baths clean perineal wounds and reduce inflammation and pain. Circulation in the perineal area is increased. Voiding may be stimulated by a sitz bath. Clients with perineal swelling (such as hemorrhoids), or perineal wounds (such as those that occur during childbirth), may be ordered to take sitz baths. Because the sitz bath causes increased blood flow to the pelvic area, blood flow to other parts of the body is decreased. Clients may feel weak, faint, or dizzy after taking a sitz bath.

Preparing and applying warm compresses

Equipment: washcloth, plastic wrap, towel, basin, bath thermometer

1 Wash your hands.

2 Explain the procedure to the client. Speak clearly, slowly, and directly. Maintain face-to-face contact whenever possible.

3 Provide privacy for the client.

4 Fill basin one-half to two-thirds full with hot water. Test water temperature with thermometer or your wrist and ensure it is safe. Water temperature should be 105° to 115°F. Have client check water temperature. Adjust if necessary.

5 Soak the washcloth in the water and wring it out. Immediately apply it to the area needing a warm compress. Note the time. Quickly cover the washcloth with plastic wrap and the towel to keep it warm.

6 Check the area every five minutes. Remove the compress if the area is red or numb or if the client complains of pain or discomfort. Change the compress if cooling occurs. Remove the compress after 20 minutes.

7 Commercial warm compresses are also available. If these are provided, follow the package directions and your supervisor's instructions.

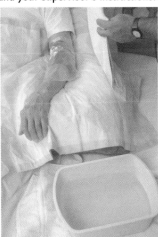

8 Discard water in the toilet. Clean and store basin and other supplies. Put laundry in hamper. Discard plastic wrap.

9 Wash your hands.

10 Document the time, length, and site of procedure, and any observations.

Administering warm soaks

Equipment: basin or bathtub (depending on the area to be soaked) bath thermometer, bath blanket, towel

1   Wash your hands.

2   Explain the procedure to the client. Speak clearly, slowly, and directly. Maintain face-to-face contact whenever possible.

3   Provide privacy for the client.

4   Fill the basin or tub half full of warm water. Test water temperature with thermometer or your wrist and ensure it is safe. Water temperature should be 105° to 110°F. Have client check water temperature. Adjust if necessary.

5   Immerse the body part in the basin, or help the client into the tub. Pad the edge of the basin with a towel if needed. Use a bath blanket to cover the rest of the client if needed for extra warmth.

6   Check water temperature every five minutes. Add hot water as needed to maintain the temperature. Never add water hotter than

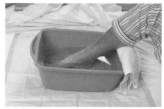

110°F to avoid burns. To prevent burns, tell the client not to add hot water him- or herself. Observe the area for redness. Discontinue the soak if the client complains of pain or discomfort.

7   Soak for 15-20 minutes, or as ordered in the care plan.

8   Remove basin or help the client out of the tub. Use the towel to dry client.

9   Drain the tub or discard water. Clean and store basin and other supplies. Put laundry in hamper.

10 Wash your hands.

11 Document the time, length, and site of procedure. Report the client's response and any of your observations about the skin.

Assisting with a sitz bath

A disposable sitz bath fits on the toilet seat and is attached to a rubber bag containing warm water.

Equipment: disposable sitz bath, bath thermometer, towels, gloves

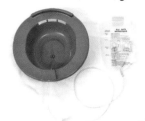

1   Wash your hands.

2   Explain the procedure to the client. Speak clearly, slowly, and

directly. Maintain face-to-face contact whenever possible.

3   Provide privacy for the client.

4   Put on gloves.

5   Fill the sitz bath two-thirds full with hot water. Place the disposable sitz bath on the toilet seat. If the sitz bath is prescribed for cleaning the perineal area, the temperature should be 100°F to 104°F. For a sitz bath given for pain and to stimulate circulation, the water temperature should be 105°F to 110°F. Check the water temperature using the bath thermometer.

6   Help the client undress and be seated on the sitz bath. A valve on

the tubing connected to the bag allows the client or you to replenish the water in the sitz bath with hot water.

7 Leave the room, but check on the client every five minutes to make sure he or she is not dizzy or weak. Stay with a client who seems unsteady.

8 Assist the client out of the sitz

bath in 20 minutes. Provide towels and help with dressing if needed.

9 Clean and store supplies.

10 Remove gloves.

11 Wash your hands.

12 Document the procedure, including the time started and ended, the client's response, and the water temperature.

Applying ice packs

Equipment: ice pack or sealable plastic bag and crushed ice, towel to cover pack or bag

1 Wash your hands.

2 Explain the procedure to the client. Speak clearly, slowly, and directly. Maintain face-to-face contact whenever possible.

3 Provide privacy for the client.

4 Fill plastic bag or ice pack one-half to two-thirds full with crushed ice. Remove excess air. Cover bag or ice pack with towel.

5 Apply bag to the area as ordered. Note the time. Use another towel to cover bag if it is too cold.

6 Check the area after ten minutes for blisters, pale, white, or gray

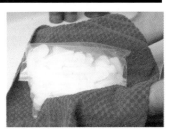

skin. Stop treatment if client complains of numbness or pain.

7 Remove ice after 20 minutes or as ordered in the care plan.

8 Return ice bag or pack to freezer.

9 Wash your hands.

10 Document the time, length, and site of procedure. Report the client's response and any of your observations about the skin.

Applying cold compresses

Equipment: basin filled with water and ice, two washcloths, plastic or rubber sheet, towels

1 Wash your hands.

2 Explain the procedure to the client. Speak clearly, slowly, and directly. Maintain face-to-face contact whenever possible.

3 Provide privacy for the client.

4 Position client on plastic sheet. Rinse washcloth in basin and wring out. Cover the area to be treated with a cloth sheet or towel. Apply cold washcloth to the area

as directed. Change washcloths often to keep area cold.

5 Check the area after five minutes for blisters, pale, white, or gray skin. Stop treatment if client complains of numbness or pain.

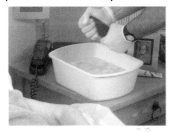

6 Remove compresses after 20 minutes or as ordered in the care plan. Give client towels as needed to dry the area.

7 Clean and store basin.

8 Wash your hands.

9 Document the time, length, and site of procedure. Report the client's response and any observations about the skin.

Medications

People who need home care often need to take several medications. HHAs do not usually handle or give medications. However, you need to understand the kinds of medicine your clients may be taking. You also need to know what to do if a client experiences side effects or refuses to take medication. If your client is taking medications that can be purchased over-the-counter (OTC) or without a physician's prescription, notify the supervisor. Sometimes OTC medications interfere with the desired effects of prescription medications.

Many states have passed different laws regarding the responsibilities and limitations for assisting clients with medications. It is very important for you to be familiar with the regulations in your state. Provide only the assistance that is allowed.

GUIDELINES: SAFE AND PROPER USE OF MEDICATIONS

- Never handle or give medications unless specifically trained and assigned to do so. Do not touch the inside of a medicine bottle or the pills or other medicines themselves. Do not put any medication in a client's mouth. Handling or giving medication can have serious consequences.

- Observe clients taking their medication. Although you cannot handle or administer medications, you can remind clients to take them. You can also bring medication containers to clients, and provide water or food as needed to take with the medication. Always observe, report, and document as appropriate.

- Know the difference between prescription drugs and over-the-counter drugs. Antiobiotics (such as penicillin), heart drugs (such as nitroglycerin), and potent pain medication (such as codeine) are examples of prescription drugs. Aspirin or cold medications, such as decongestants, are over-the-counter drugs.

- Be aware of all medications a client is taking, both prescription and nonprescription. There are many possible side effects and interactions among medications. Watch for symptoms such as itching, trembling or shaking, anxiety, stomachache, diarrhea, confusion, vomiting, constipation, loss of appetite, rash, hives, or headache. Any of these symptoms could indicate a side effect or interaction. Report any of these symptoms to your supervisor.

Knowing and remembering the five "rights" of medications will help prevent mistakes.

1 The Right Client.

2 The Right Medication.

3 The Right Time.

4 The Right Route.

5 The Right Amount.

If the medication label and the care plan do not agree on any of the five "rights," call your supervisor. Also, if there is not enough information, or if you have noticed another problem with the medication (for example, the client's name is not on the container), call your supervisor.

If a client shows signs of a bad reaction to a medication, or complains of side effects, report these right away. Your supervisor can assess whether the symptom is caused by the medication. Your responsibility is to report your observations.

MEDICATIONS: OBSERVING AND REPORTING

- dizziness, fainting

- nausea, vomiting

- rash, hives, itching

- difficulty breathing, swelling of throat or eyes

- drowsiness

- headache, blurred vision

- abdominal pain

- diarrhea or constipation

- any other unusual sign

In addition, report any of the following problems immediately:

- Client refuses to take medication as directed.

- Client takes the wrong dose (amount) of medication.

- Client takes medication at the wrong time.

- Client takes the wrong medication.
- A medication container is missing or empty.

If a client has difficulty swallowing the medication, report this to your supervisor. The doctor can then make appropriate changes. Do not crush tablets or empty capsules of medications into the client's food or drinks unless the label specifically instructs you to do so.

If a client has a severe allergic reaction to a medication, takes the wrong dose, or takes medications together that cause complications, emergency medical treatment is necessary. Treat an overdose of medication, whether it was accidental or intentional, as a poisoning. Call the local Poison Control number immediately. Follow their instructions. Poison Control will send paramedics or an ambulance if needed. For severe drug reactions or interactions, call 911 or 0 for emergency help. Stay with the client. Do not give any liquids, food, or other medications unless instructed to do so by emergency personnel. Notify your supervisor as soon as possible.

You may be required to assist with the proper storage of medications.

GUIDELINES: PROPER STORAGE OF MEDICATIONS

- Keep the client's medications in one place, separate from medicine used by other members of the household.

- If there are young children or a disoriented elderly person in the home, recommend to the family that medications be locked away.

- All medications should be kept in child-proof containers if children are in the home. To avoid an accidental overdose, keep medications out of reach of children.

- If medicine requires refrigeration, make sure the bottle is on an upper shelf in the back, out of a child's reach.

- All medications should be stored away from heat and light, as appropriate.

- The client or family member should discard medications that have expired, are not labeled, or are discolored. Make sure these medications are not discarded in the trash. Children or animals may have access to them. Ask your supervisor for specific disposal instructions if the client or family will not dispose of expired medications. Do not dispose of them yourself.

The drugs that pose the highest risk for causing drug dependency are pain medications and tranquilizers. Substance abuse refers to the use of legal or illegal drugs, cigarettes, or alcohol in a way that is harmful to oneself or others. It is not necessary for a substance to be illegal for it to be abused. Alcohol and cigarettes are legal for adults, but are often abused. Over-the-counter medications, including diet aids and decongestants, can be addictive and harmful. Even household substances such as paint or glue are increasingly abused, causing injury and death.

Possible signs of substance abuse include the following:

- changes in personality, moodiness, strange behavior, disruption of routines
- changes in physical appearance (red eyes, dilated pupils, weight loss)
- smell of cigarettes, liquor, or other substances on breath or clothes
- diminished sense of smell
- loss of appetite
- inability to function normally at school or work
- need for money, or money missing from the home
- alcohol or cigarettes missing from the home
- new friends or companions, strange phone calls

Report these signs to your supervisor. You can report your observations without accusing anyone of abuse. Simply report what you see, not what you think the cause may be.

Oxygen

Some clients with breathing difficulties may receive oxygen. It is more concentrated than what we breathe in the air. A doctor prescribes oxygen. You should never stop, adjust, or administer oxygen for a client. Oxygen will be delivered to the home in tanks or produced by an oxygen concentrator. An oxygen concentrator changes air in the room into air with more oxygen. The agency that supplies the oxygen will service the equipment and will provide training in its use.

Oxygen is a highly combustible gas. It can very easily explode or catch fire. Working around oxygen requires special safety precautions.

GUIDELINES: WORKING SAFELY AROUND OXYGEN

- Remove all fire hazards from the area. Fire hazards include electrical appliances, cigarettes, matches, and fluids that may catch fire easily. Notify your supervisor if a fire hazard is present and the client does not want it removed.

- Post "No Smoking" and "Oxygen in Use" signs. Never allow smoking in the room or area where oxygen is used or stored.

- Never allow candles or other open flames around oxygen.

- Learn how to turn oxygen off in case of fire. Never adjust oxygen level.

- Report if the nasal cannula or face mask is causing skin irritation. Check behind the ears for irritation from the nasal cannula.

IVs

IV stands for intravenous (in-tra-VEE-nus), or into a vein. A client with an IV is receiving medication, nutrition, or fluids through a vein. When a physician prescribes an IV, a nurse inserts a needle into a vein. This allows direct access to the bloodstream. Medication, nutrition, or fluids either drip from a bag suspended on a pole or are pumped by a portable pump through a tube and into the vein. Some clients with chronic conditions may have a permanent opening for IVs. This opening has been surgically created to allow easy access for IV fluids.

HHAs never insert or remove IV lines. You will not be responsible for care of the site. Your only responsibility for IV care is to report and document any observations of changes or problems with the IV.

IVS: OBSERVING AND REPORTING

- the needle falls out or is removed

- the dressing around the IV site is loose or not intact

- blood is visible in the tubing or around the site of the IV

- the site is swollen or discolored

- the client complains of pain

- the bag is broken, or the level of fluid does not seem to decrease

- the IV fluid is not dripping

- the IV fluid is nearly gone

- the pump beeps, indicating a problem

- the pump is dropped

V
Special Clients, Special Needs

15. Disabilities and Mental Illnesses

Guidelines for Disabilities

A disability is the impairment of a physical or mental function. Disability may result from a disease, a complication of pregnancy, or an injury. Depending on the disability, a person may not be able to perform activities of daily living (ADLs). Work and social activities may be limited. People with disabilities may be more susceptible to illness. By strictly following the client care plan and carefully observing and reporting, you can help your clients with disabilities avoid illness. Your efforts may also help clients lead more independent lives.

Families of people with disabilities may find it difficult to cope with the stress a disability can cause. They may feel resentment, disappointment, guilt or shame, and anger or frustration. Caring for someone with a disability can be a big responsibility. It affects a family's time, energy, patience, and financial resources. Home health aides can give family members a much-needed break. Clients and their families may need additional support, possibly including counseling, to help deal with the disability. Tell your supervisor if you think a client or family member needs additional support to cope with a disability.

Illness or disability requires clients and families to make adjustments. Making these adjustments may be difficult, depending on the family's emotional, spiritual, and financial resources. Some of the personal adjustments include the following:

- accepting the illness or disability and its long-term consequences
- finding money to pay expenses of hospitalization or home care
- dealing with paperwork required for insurance, Medicaid, or Medicare
- taking care of tasks the client can no longer handle

- understanding medical information and making difficult care decisions
- providing daily care when the aide cannot be there

GUIDELINES: WORKING WITH DISABILITIES

- Promote self care and independence.
- Assure the client's safety.
- Promote the client's health and comfort.
- Maintain the client's dignity and self-worth.
- Maintain the stability of the client's household.

When asked what qualities they need and value most in home care workers, people with disabilities list the following:

1 Punctuality

2 Reliability

3 Responsiveness to needs

4 Continuity

5 Positive attitude

Guidelines for Mental Illnesses

Mental health is the normal functioning of emotional and intellectual abilities. Characteristics of a person who is mentally healthy include the abilities to:

- get along with others
- adapt to change, care for self and others, and give and accept love
- deal with situations that cause anxiety, disappointment, and frustration
- take responsibility for decisions, feelings, and actions
- control and fulfill desires and impulses appropriately

Although it involves the emotions and mental functions, mental illness is a disease. It is similar to any physical disease. It produces signs and symptoms and affects the body's ability to function. It responds to proper treatment and care. Mental illness disrupts a person's ability to function at a normal level in the family, home, or community. It often produces inappropriate behavior. Some signs and symptoms of mental illness include confusion, disorientation, agitation, and anxiety.

Mental illness can be caused or made worse by chronic stress from any of the following conditions:

- physical factors, such as illness, disability, or aging
- substance abuse or a chemical imbalance
- environmental factors, such as weak interpersonal or family relationships or traumatic early life experiences
- heredity
- stress

Mentally healthy people are able to control their emotions and their responses. Mentally ill people usually do not have this control. Knowing mental illness is a disease helps you work with mentally ill clients. Mental health is important to physical health. The ability of mentally healthy people to reduce stress can help prevent some physical illnesses. It can help them cope if illness or disability occur. Mental health can help protect and improve physical health. The reverse is also true. Physical illness or disability can cause or worsen mental illness. The stress these conditions create takes a toll on mental health.

Different types of mental illness will determine how well clients are able to communicate. Treat each client as an individual.

GUIDELINES: COMMUNICATING WITH CLIENTS WHO ARE MENTALLY ILL

- Do not talk to adults as if they were children.
- Use simple, clear statements and a normal tone of voice.
- Be sure that what you say and how you say it show respect and concern.
- Sit or stand at a normal distance from the client. Be aware of your body language.
- Be honest and straightforward, as you would with any client.
- Avoid arguments.
- Maintain eye contact.
- Listen carefully.

There are many degrees of mental illness, from mild to severe. Being able to recognize some behaviors may make it easier to understand mentally ill clients:

Anxiety-Related Disorders. Anxiety (ang-ZYE-i-tee) is uneasiness or fear, often about a situation or condition. Physical symptoms of anxiety-related disorders include shakiness, muscle aches, sweating, cold and clammy hands, dizziness, fatigue, racing heart, cold or hot flashes, a choking or smothering sensation, or a dry mouth.

Phobias (FOH-bee-uhs) are an intense form of anxiety. Many people are intensely afraid of certain things (for example, dogs or snakes) or situations (like being in a confined space, or flying). For a mentally ill person, a phobia is a disabling terror. It prevents the person from participating in normal activities.

Panic disorder causes a person to be terrified for no apparent reason.

Obsessive compulsive disorder is the name for obsessive behavior a person uses to cope with anxiety. For example, a person may wash his hands over and over again as a way of dealing with guilt.

Anxiety-related disorders may also be caused by a traumatic experience. This type of anxiety is known as **post-traumatic stress disorder**.

Depression. Clinical depression is a serious mental illness that may cause intense mental, emotional, and physical pain and disability.

Symptoms of people who are clinically depressed include the following:

- pain, including headaches, abdominal pain, and other body aches
- low energy or fatigue
- apathy, or lack of interest in activities
- irritability
- anxiety
- problems with sexual functioning and desire
- sleeplessness, difficulty sleeping, or excessive sleeping
- guilt
- difficulty concentrating
- recurrent thoughts of suicide and death

Schizophrenia (skit-zo-FRAY-nee-a). Contrary to popular belief, schizophrenia does not mean "split personality." Schizophrenia is a brain disorder that affects a person's ability to think and communicate clearly. It also affects the ability to manage emotions, make decisions, and understand reality. Some of the symptoms of schizophrenia are:

- hallucinations

- delusions

- disorganized thinking and speech

- person moves slowly, repeating rhythmic gestures or movements

- person may also show less emotion, less interest in the things around them

- lack of energy

Mental illness can be treated. Medication and psychotherapy are common treatment methods. Medication can have a very positive effect. It may allow mentally ill people to function more completely. As with all medication, drugs used to treat mental illness must be taken properly to promote benefits and reduce side effects. Home health aides may be assigned to observe clients taking their medications.

GUIDELINES: PERSONAL CARE OF MENTALLY ILL CLIENTS

- Follow the care plan to tell you what kinds of care and what procedures you must perform.

- Support the client and the family.

- Be positive and professional with the client and the family.

- Encourage clients to do as much for themselves as possible. Be patient and supportive.

MENTALLY ILL CLIENTS: OBSERVING AND REPORTING

- changes in ability

- positive or negative mood changes, especially withdrawal

- behavior changes, including changes in personality, extreme behavior, and behavior that does not seem appropriate to the situation

- comments, even jokes, about hurting self or others

- failure to take medicine or improper use of medicine

- real or imagined physical symptoms

- events, situations, or people that seem to upset or excite clients

16. Special Conditions

There are certain special conditions or diseases you will see in the home that require special and specific types of care. Below is a quick overview of these special conditions for you to use as a reference when you care for clients with any of the following conditions:

- Arthritis
- Cancer
- Diabetes
- Cerebral Vascular Accident or Stroke
- Circulatory Disorders
- HIV/AIDS
- Dementia
- Alzheimer's Disease
- Chronic Obstructive Pulmonary Disease (COPD)
- Hip/Knee Replacement

Arthritis

Arthritis is a general term that refers to inflammation, or swelling, of the joints. It causes stiffness, pain, and decreased mobility. Arthritis may be the result of aging, injury, or an autoimmune illness. During an autoimmune illness, the body's immune system attacks normal tissue in the body. There are several types of arthritis.

1 **Osteoarthritis** (AH-stee-oh-ar-thrye-tis). Osteoarthritis is a common type of arthritis that affects the elderly. It may occur with aging or as the result of joint injury.

   - Hips and knees, which are weight-bearing joints, are usually affected. Joints of the fingers, thumbs, and spine can also be affected.

   - Pain and stiffness seem to increase in cold or damp weather.

2 **Rheumatoid Arthritis** (ROOM-a-toyd ar-THRYE-tis). Rheumatoid arthritis can affect people of all ages.

   - Joints become inflamed, red, swollen, and very painful. Movement is eventually restricted.

   - Fever, fatigue, and weight loss are also symptoms.

Arthritis is generally treated with some or all of the following:

- anti-inflammatory medications such as aspirin or ibuprofen
- local applications of heat to reduce swelling and pain
- range of motion exercises

- a regular exercise and/or activity regimen
- diet to reduce weight or maintain strength

GUIDELINES: CARING FOR CLIENTS WITH ARTHRITIS

- Watch for stomach irritation or heartburn caused by aspirin or ibuprofen. Some clients cannot take these medications. Report signs of stomach irritation immediately.

- Encourage activity. Gentle activity can help reduce the effects of arthritis. Follow the care plan instructions carefully. Use canes or other walking aids as needed.

- Adapt activities of daily living (ADLs) to allow independence. Many devices are available to allow clients to bathe, dress, and feed themselves even when they have arthritis.

- Choose clothing that is easy to put on and fasten. Suggest handrails and safety bars for the bathroom. Special utensils are available to make it easier for clients to feed themselves.

- Treat each client as an individual. Arthritis is very common among elderly clients. Do not assume that all clients have the same symptoms and need the same care.

- Help maintain client's self-esteem by encouraging self care. Maintain a positive attitude. Listen to the client's feelings.

Cancer

Cancer is a general term used to describe many types of malignant tumors. A tumor is a cluster of abnormally growing cells. Benign tumors grow slowly in local areas. They are considered noncancerous. Malignant tumors grow rapidly and invade surrounding tissues.

Cancer invades local tissue, and it can spread to other parts of the body. When cancer spreads from the site where it first appears, it can affect one or more other body systems. In general, treatment is more difficult and cancer is more deadly after this has occurred. Cancer often appears first in the breast, colon, rectum, uterus, prostate, lungs, or skin.

Risk factors for cancer include the following:

- tobacco use
- exposure to sunlight
- excessive alcohol use
- exposure to some chemicals and industrial agents

- some food additives
- radiation
- poor nutrition
- lack of physical activity

When diagnosed early, cancer can often be treated and controlled. The American Cancer Society has identified seven warning signs of cancer:

1 Change in bowel or bladder habits

2 A sore that does not heal

3 Unusual bleeding or discharge from a body opening

4 Thickening or lump in the breast or elsewhere

5 Indigestion or difficulty swallowing

6 Obvious change in a wart or mole

7 Nagging cough or persistent hoarseness

People with cancer can often live longer and sometimes recover if they are treated early. Treatments include:

- surgery
- chemotherapy
- radiation

GUIDELINES: CARING FOR CLIENTS WITH CANCER

- Each case is different. Cancer is a general term and refers to many separate situations. Clients may expect to live many years or only several months.

- Treatment affects each person differently. Do not make assumptions about a client's condition.

- Clients may want to talk or may avoid talking. Respect each client's needs.

- Be honest. Never tell a client, "everything will be okay."

- Be sensitive. Remember that cancer is a disease, and we do not know its cause.

- Good nutrition is extremely important for clients with cancer. Follow the care plan instructions carefully. Use plastic utensils for a client receiving chemotherapy. Metal utensils can cause a bitter taste.

- Cancer can cause terrible pain, especially in the late stages. Watch your client for signs of pain. Assist with comfort measures, including repositioning and providing distractions such as conversation, music, or reading materials.

- Use lotion regularly on dry or delicate skin. Do not apply lotion to areas receiving radiation therapy.

- Offer back rubs to provide comfort and increase circulation.

- Help clients brush and floss teeth regularly. Medications, nausea, vomiting, or mouth infections may cause a bad taste in the mouth. Use a soft-bristled toothbrush and rinse with baking soda and water or a prescribed rinse.

- People with cancer may suffer from a low self-image because they are weak and their appearance has changed. For example, hair loss is a common side effect of chemotherapy. Assist with grooming if desired.

- If visitors help cheer your client, encourage them and do not intrude. If some times of day are better than others, suggest this to the client's friends and family.

- Caring for a person with cancer at home can be very difficult for family members. Be alert to needs that are not being met or stresses created by the illness. Report your observations.

Numerous services and support groups are available for people with cancer and their families or caregivers. Hospitals, hospice programs, churches, and synagogues offer many resources, including meal services, transportation to doctors' offices or hospitals, counseling, and support groups. Check the local yellow pages under "cancer," or call the local or state chapter of the American Cancer Society. You can also contact your local Area Agency on Aging.

Diabetes

In diabetes mellitus, commonly called diabetes, the pancreas does not produce enough insulin. Insulin is the substance the body needs to convert glucose (GLOO-kohs), or natural sugar, into energy for the body. Without insulin to process the glucose, these sugars collect in the blood. This causes problems with circulation and can damage vital organs. Diabetes commonly occurs in people with a family history of the illness, in the elderly, and in people who are obese. Two types of diabetes have been identified:

1 Type 1 is usually diagnosed in children and young adults. It was formerly known as juvenile diabetes. It most often appears before age 20. In Type 1 diabetes, the body does not produce insulin. This condition will continue throughout a person's life. A person can develop

Type 1 diabetes up to age 40. Type 1 diabetes is treated with insulin and a special diet.

2 Type 2 diabetes is the most common form of diabetes. In Type 2 diabetes, either the body does not produce enough insulin or the body fails to properly use insulin. This is known as "insulin resistance." It can usually be controlled with diet and/or oral medications. This type is also called adult-onset diabetes. Type 2 diabetes usually develops slowly. It is the milder form of diabetes. It typically develops around age 35. Type 2 diabetes often occurs in obese people or those with a family history of the disease.

People with diabetes mellitus may have these signs and symptoms:

- increased thirst
- increased hunger
- weight loss
- elevated levels of blood sugar
- presence of sugar in the urine
- increased frequency of urination

Diabetes can lead to the following complications:

- Changes in the circulatory system can cause heart attack and stroke, reduced circulation, poor wound healing, and kidney and nerve damage.
- Damage to the eyes can cause vision loss and blindness.
- Poor circulation and impaired wound healing may cause leg and foot ulcers, infected wounds, and gangrene. Gangrene can lead to amputation.

Insulin shock and diabetic coma are complications of diabetes that can be life-threatening. Refer to the Medical Emergencies section for more information on insulin shock and diabetic coma. Discuss each individual client's status with your supervisor.

Diabetes must be carefully controlled to prevent complications and severe illness. When working with clients with diabetes, follow care plan instructions carefully.

GUIDELINES: CARING FOR CLIENTS WITH DIABETES

- Follow diet instructions exactly. The intake of carbohydrates, including breads, potatoes, grains, pasta, and sugars, must be regulated. Meals must be eaten at the same time each day. The client must eat everything that is served. If a client refuses to eat what is directed, or if you suspect that he or she is not following the diet when you leave, report this to your supervisor.

- Encourage your client to follow his exercise program. A regular exercise program is important. It affects how quickly our bodies use the food we eat. Exercise also helps improve circulation. Exercises may include walking or other active exercise. It may also include passive range of motion exercises. Assist with exercises as necessary.

- Observe the client's management of insulin doses. Doses are calculated exactly. They should be administered at the same time each day. Home health aides are not permitted to inject insulin.

- Perform urine and blood tests as directed. Sometimes the care plan will specify a daily blood or urine test to determine sugar or insulin levels. Not all states allow home health aides to do this. Know your state's rules. Your agency will train you.

- Perform foot care only as directed. Because poor circulation occurs in diabetics, even a small sore on the leg or foot can grow into a large wound. It can result in amputation. Careful foot care, including regular inspection, is very important. The goals of diabetic foot care are to check for signs of irritation or sores, to promote blood circulation, and to prevent infection.

Providing foot care for the diabetic client

Equipment: basin of warm water, mild soap, washcloth, soft towel, lotion, cotton balls, cotton socks, shoes or slippers, gloves if client has broken skin

1 Wash your hands.

2 Explain the procedure to the client. Speak clearly, slowly, and directly. Maintain face-to-face contact whenever possible.

3 Provide privacy for the client.

4 Put on gloves if the client has broken skin.

5 Using the washcloth and soap, wash the feet gently. Rinse with the warm water.

6 Pat the feet dry gently, wiping between the toes.

7 Starting at the toes and working up to the ankles, gently rub lotion into the feet with circular strokes. Your goal is to increase circulation, so take several minutes on each foot.

8 Observe the feet, ankles, and legs for dry skin, irritation, blisters, redness, sores, corns, discoloration, or swelling.

9 Help client put on socks and shoes or slippers.

10 Put used linens in the laundry. Pour water into the toilet. Clean and store basin and supplies.

11 Remove gloves if worn.

12 Wash your hands.

13 Document the procedure, including any abnormalities you observed on the feet or legs.

In addition to daily foot care, encourage diabetic clients to wear comfortable, well-fitting shoes that do not hurt their feet. To avoid cuts or injuries to the feet, diabetics should never go barefoot. Cotton socks are best because they absorb sweat. Home health aides should never trim or clip any client's toenails, but especially not a diabetic client's toenails. Only a nurse or doctor should trim a diabetic's toenails.

People with diabetes must be very careful about what they eat. To keep their blood glucose levels near normal, they must eat the right amount of the right type of food at the right time. To make it easier to keep track of what they should eat, diabetics often follow meal plans and use exchange lists.

A dietitian, working with the client, creates a meal plan that includes all the right types and amounts of food for each day. Then the client uses exchange lists, or lists of similar foods that can substitute for one another, to make up a menu. For example, the meal plan might call for one starch and one fruit to be eaten as a snack. Looking at the exchange list, the client may choose which starch and fruit he wants to eat. The equivalent serving size for each food is also given, so the person will get the right amount of carbohydrates, protein, and fat to meet his or her requirements. Using meal plans and exchange lists, a person with diabetes can control his diet while still making his own food choices. Refer to the "Special Diets" section in Section VI for more information.

CVA or Stroke

The medical term for a stroke is a cerebral vascular accident (CVA). CVA, or stroke, is caused when blood supply to the brain is cut off suddenly by a clot or a ruptured blood vessel. Without blood, part of the brain gets no oxygen. This causes brain cells to die. Refer to the Medical Emergencies section for more information on the warning signs of a stroke.

The two sides of the brain control different functions. Symptoms depend on which side of the brain the stroke affected. Weaknesses on the right side of the body indicate that the left side of the brain was affected. Weaknesses on the left side of the body indicate that the right side of the brain was affected.

Strokes can be mild or severe. After a stroke, a client may experience any of the following:

- weakness or paralysis on one side of the body
- difficulty speaking or inability to speak

- difficulty understanding spoken or written words

- loss of sensations such as temperature or touch

- loss of bowel or bladder control

- confusion

- poor judgment

- memory loss

- loss of cognitive abilities

- tendency to ignore one side of the body

- difficulty swallowing

If the stroke was mild, the client may experience few, if any, of these effects. Physical therapy may help stroke victims regain physical abilities. Speech therapy and occupational therapy can also help a person learn to communicate and perform ADLs again.

GUIDELINES: CARING FOR CLIENTS RECOVERING FROM STROKE

- Clients with paralysis, weakness, or loss of movement will usually receive physical therapy or occupational therapy. You may be asked to assist clients in performing exercises.

- Clients may also need to perform leg exercises to improve circulation. Safety is important when post-CVA clients are exercising.

- Adapt procedures when providing personal care for clients with one-sided paralysis or weakness.

- When helping with transfers or walking, stand on the weaker side. Always use a gait belt for safety.

- Never refer to the weaker side as the "bad side," or talk about the "bad" leg or arm. Use the terms "weaker," "affected," or "involved" to refer to the side with paralysis or paresis.

- Clients with speech loss or communication problems may receive speech therapy. You may be asked to help. This includes helping clients to recognize written words or to speak words.

- Use verbal and nonverbal communication to express your positive attitude. Let the client know you have confidence in his or her abilities through smiles, touches, and gestures.

Experiencing confusion or memory loss is upsetting. People often cry for no apparent reason after suffering a stroke. Be patient and understanding. Keeping a routine may help clients feel more secure.

Monitoring the home safety of clients who have had a stroke is essential. Clients who are unsteady, weak, or confused are at risk of falling. Clients with loss of sensation are at risk of burning themselves in the bathroom or at the stove. Some safety tips include:

- Remove any hazards from the home, including unnecessary clutter or throw rugs.

- Unplug appliances like toasters and coffee makers when not in use.

- Check the refrigerator and cabinets for spoiled food. A stroke may impair the senses of smell and taste.

- Report any suspected safety hazards to your supervisor.

- Follow instructions for safe client transfers using good body mechanics.

- Always check on the client's body alignment. Sometimes an arm or leg can be caught and the client is unaware.

- Pay special attention to skin care and observing for changes in the skin if a client is unable to move.

Some important ways HHAs can assist the client recovering from stroke are:

- Encourage independence and self-esteem. Let the client do things for himself whenever possible, even if you could do a better or faster job.

- Appreciate and acknowledge clients' efforts to do things for themselves even when they are unsuccessful.

- Praise even the smallest successes to build confidence.

GUIDELINES: TRANSFERRING THE CLIENT WITH ONE-SIDED WEAKNESS

- Support the involved side.

- Lead with the uninvolved (stronger) side.

- Follow the principles of good body mechanics.

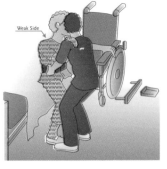

GUIDELINES: DRESSING A CLIENT WITH ONE-SIDED WEAKNESS

- Dress weaker side first. Place the weaker arm or leg into the clothing first. This prevents unnecessary bending and stretching of the limb. Undress stronger side first. Lead with the stronger side. Then remove the weaker arm or leg from clothing to prevent the limb from being stretched and twisted.

- Use adaptive equipment to help client dress himself.
- Encourage self-care.

GUIDELINES: ASSISTING A CLIENT WITH EATING

- Be sure to place food in the client's field of vision. Use assistive devices such as silverware with built-up handle grips, plate guards, and drinking cups.
- Watch for signs of choking.
- Serve soft foods if swallowing is difficult.

Depending on the severity of the stroke and speech loss or confusion, the following tips may be helpful:

- Keep your questions and directions simple.
- Phrase questions so they can be answered with a "yes" or "no."
- Agree on signals, such as shaking or nodding the head, or raising a hand or finger to indicate "yes" or "no."
- Use pictures, gestures, or pointing. Use communication boards or special cards to make communication easier.
- Use a pencil and paper if a client is able to write. A thick handle or tape wrapped around the pen may help the client hold it more easily.
- Keep a bell or other call signal within reach of clients. They can let you know when you are needed.
- Never talk about a client as if he or she were not there. Speak to all clients with respect.

Circulatory Disorders

Hypertension or High Blood Pressure

When blood pressure consistently measures higher than 140/90, a person is diagnosed as having hypertension, or high blood pressure. If blood pressure is between 120/80 and 139/89 mmHg, it is called prehypertension. This means that person does not have high blood pressure now but is likely to develop it in the future. Hypertension is caused by atherosclerosis (ath-er-oh-skle-ROH-sis), or a hardening and narrowing of the blood vessels. It can also result from kidney disease, tumors of the adrenal gland, complications of pregnancy, and head injuries. Hypertension can develop in persons of any age.

Signs and symptoms of hypertension are not always obvious, especially in the early stages. Often it is only discovered when a blood pressure measurement is taken. Persons with the disease may complain of headache, blurred vision, and dizziness.

GUIDELINES: CARING FOR CLIENTS WITH HYPERTENSION

- Because it can lead to serious conditions such as CVA, heart attack, kidney disease, or blindness, treatment to control high blood pressure is essential. Clients may take medication that lowers cholesterol or diuretics. Diuretics are drugs that reduce fluid in the body.

- Clients may also have a prescribed exercise program or be on a special low-fat, low-sodium diet.

Coronary Artery Disease (CAD)

Coronary artery disease occurs when the blood vessels in the coronary arteries narrow. This reduces the supply of blood to the heart muscle and deprives it of oxygen and nutrients. Over time, as fatty deposits block the artery, the muscle that was supplied by the blood vessel dies. CAD can lead to heart attack or stroke.

The heart muscle that is not getting enough oxygen causes chest pain, or angina pectoris. The heart needs more oxygen during exercise or exertion, stress, excitement, or a heavy meal. In CAD, constricted blood vessels prevent the extra blood with oxygen from getting to the heart.

The pain of angina pectoris is usually described as pressure or tightness in the left side of the chest or in the center of the chest behind the sternum or breastbone. Some people complain of the pain radiating or extending down the inside of the left arm or to the neck and left side of the jaw. A person suffering from angina pectoris may perspire or appear pale. The person may feel dizzy and have difficulty breathing.

GUIDELINES: CARING FOR CLIENTS WITH ANGINA PECTORIS

- Rest is extremely important. Rest reduces the heart's need for extra oxygen. It helps the blood flow return to normal, often within three to fifteen minutes.

- Medication is also necessary to relax the walls of the coronary arteries. This allows them to dilate or open to allow increased blood flow to the heart muscle. This medication, nitroglycerin (nite-ro-GLIS-er-in), is a small tablet that the client places under the tongue. There it is dissolved and rapidly absorbed. Clients who have angina pectoris should keep nitroglycerin at hand to use as soon as symptoms arise.

- Clients may also be required to avoid heavy meals, overeating, intense exercise, and exposure to cold or hot and humid weather.

Myocardial Infarction (MI) or Heart Attack

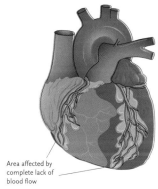

When blood flow to the heart muscle is completely blocked, oxygen and important nutrients fail to reach the cells in that region. Waste products are not removed and the muscle cell dies. This is called a myocardial infarction (MI), or heart attack. The area of dead tissue may be large or small, depending on the artery involved. Refer to the Medical Emergencies section for more information on signs and symptoms of MI.

Area affected by complete lack of blood flow

GUIDELINES: CARING FOR CLIENTS RECOVERING FROM HEART ATTACKS

- Generally clients will be placed on a regular exercise program.

- Clients may be on a diet that is low in fat and cholesterol and/or a low-sodium diet.

- Medications may be prescribed to regulate heart rate and blood pressure.

- Clients may be cautioned to avoid exposure to cold temperatures.

Congestive Heart Failure (CHF)

Coronary artery disease, heart attack, hypertension, or other disorders may all damage the heart. When the heart muscle has been severely damaged, the heart fails to pump effectively. Blood backs up into the heart instead of circulating. This is called congestive heart failure, or CHF. It can occur on one or both sides of the heart.

CONGESTIVE HEART FAILURE: OBSERVING AND REPORTING

- difficulty breathing; coughing or gurgling with breathing

- dizziness, confusion, and fainting

- pale or bluish skin

- low blood pressure

- swelling of the feet and ankles

- bulging veins in the neck

- weight gain

GUIDELINES: CARING FOR CLIENTS WITH CONGESTIVE HEART FAILURE

- Medications can strengthen the heart muscle and improve its pumping.

- Medications help eliminate excess fluids. This means more frequent trips to the bathroom. Assist clients as needed.

- A low-sodium diet may be recommended.

- Intake of fluids and output of urine may need to be measured.

- Client may weigh daily at the same time to note weight gain from fluid retention.

- Elastic leg stockings may be applied to reduce swelling in feet and ankles.

- Range of motion exercises can improve muscle tone when activity and exercise are limited.

- Assistance with personal care and ADLs may need to be provided.

HIV/AIDS

Acquired immune deficiency syndrome (AIDS) is caused by the human immunodeficiency virus (HIV). HIV attacks the body's immune system and gradually disables it. Eventually the HIV-infected person has weakened resistance to other infections. Death is the result of these infections. HIV is a sexually-transmitted disease. It is also spread through blood, infected needles, or to the fetus from its mother.

In general, HIV affects the body in stages. The first stage involves symptoms similar to flu, with fever, muscle aches, cough, and fatigue. These are signs of the immune system fighting the infection. As the infection worsens, the immune system overreacts. It attacks not only the virus, but also normal tissue.

When the virus weakens the immune system in later stages, a group of problems may appear. These include infections, tumors, and central nervous system symptoms. These problems would not occur if the immune system were healthy. This stage of the disease is known as AIDS.

In the late stages of AIDS, damage to the central nervous system may cause memory loss, poor coordination, paralysis, and confusion. These symptoms together are known as AIDS dementia complex.

The following are the signs and symptoms of HIV infection and AIDS:

- appetite loss
- involuntary weight loss of ten pounds or more
- vague, flu-like symptoms, including fever, cough, weakness, and severe or constant fatigue
- night sweats
- swollen lymph nodes in the neck, underarms, or groin
- severe diarrhea
- dry cough
- skin rashes
- painful white spots in the mouth or on the tongue
- cold sores or fever blisters on the lips and flat, white ulcers on a reddened base in the mouth
- cauliflower-like warts on the skin and in the mouth
- inflamed and bleeding gums
- bruising that does not go away
- low resistance to infection, particularly pneumonia, but also tuberculosis, herpes, bacterial infections, and hepatitis
- Kaposi's sarcoma, a form of skin cancer that appears as purple or red skin lesions
- pneumocystis pneumonia (new-moh-SIS-tis new-MOH-nee-a), a lung infection
- AIDS dementia complex

Infections, such as pneumonia, tuberculosis, and hepatitis, invade the body when the immune system is weak and cannot defend itself. These illnesses complicate AIDS. They further weaken the immune system. It is difficult to treat these infections because generally, over time, a person develops resistance to some antibiotics. These infections are frequently the cause of death in people with AIDS.

Persons who are infected with HIV are treated with drugs that slow the progress of the disease, but do not cure it. The medicines must be taken at precise times. They have many unpleasant side effects. For some people, the medications work less well than for others. Other aspects of HIV treatment include relief of symptoms and prevention and treatment of infection. You can help prevent the spread of HIV/AIDS by carefully following Standard Precautions.

You can provide valuable care for your clients who have HIV or AIDS. Their care will focus on the relief of symptoms and prevention of complications.

GUIDELINES: CARING FOR CLIENTS WITH HIV/AIDS

- Involuntary weight loss occurs in almost all people who develop AIDS. High-protein, high-calorie, and high-nutrient meals and supplements can help maintain a healthy weight.

- Some people with HIV/AIDS lose their appetites and have difficulty eating. Serve familiar and favorite foods in a pleasant setting.

- Carefully follow guidelines for safe food preparation and storage when working with a client who has HIV/AIDS. Food-borne illnesses caused by improperly cooking or storing food can cause death for someone with HIV/AIDS.

- Wash your hands frequently. Keep everything clean (especially countertops, cutting boards, and knives after they have been used to cut meat). Thaw food in the refrigerator, and wash and cook foods thoroughly. When storing food, keep cold foods cold and hot foods hot. Use small containers that seal tightly. Check expiration dates, and remember "when in doubt, throw it out."

- Clients who have infections of the mouth and esophagus may require food that is low in acid and neither cold nor hot. Spicy seasonings should be removed. Soft or pureed foods may be easier to swallow. Drinking liquid meals and fortified drinks, such as milk shakes, may ease the pain of chewing. Warm salt water or other rinses may help painful sores of the mouth. Good mouth care is essential.

- Someone who has nausea or vomiting should eat small, frequent meals, if possible. The person should eat slowly. The person should avoid high-fat and spicy foods, and eat a soft, bland diet. This includes mashed potatoes, noodles, rice, crackers, pretzels, toast, gelatin, and clear soups. Cold foods that have little odor are usually easier to eat than hot foods. When nausea and vomiting persist, liquids and salty foods should be encouraged. These include clear soups, clear juices, ginger ale and colas, saltines, and pretzels. Clients should eat small, frequent meals and drink fluids in between meals. Care must be taken to maintain an adequate intake of fluids.

- Clients who have mild diarrhea may have frequent small meals that are low in fat, fiber, and milk products. If diarrhea is severe, the client's doctor may order a "BRAT" diet (a diet consisting of bananas, rice, apples, and toast). This diet is helpful for short-term use.

- Neuropathy (NOOR-oh-path-ee), or numbness, tingling, and pain in the feet and legs is usually treated with pain medications. Going without shoes or wearing loose, soft slippers may be helpful. If blankets and sheets cause pain, use a bed cradle to keep sheets and blankets from resting on the legs and feet.

- Clients with HIV/AIDS may suffer from anxiety and depression. In addition, they often suffer the judgments of family, friends, and society. Some people may blame them for their illness. People with HIV/AIDS may experience tremendous stress. They may feel uncertainty about their illness, health care, and finances. They may also have lost people in their social support network of friends and family.

- Clients with HIV/AIDS need support from others. This support may come from family, friends, religious and community groups, and support groups, as well as the healthcare team. Treat all your clients with respect and help provide the emotional support they need.

Withdrawal, apathy, avoidance of complex tasks, and mental slowness are symptoms that appear early in HIV infection. In addition, medications may cause side effects of this type. Later, AIDS dementia complex may develop, causing further mental symptoms. There may also be muscle weakness and loss of muscle control, making falls a risk. Clients in this stage of the disease will need a safe environment and close supervision in their ADLs.

Dementia

As we age, we may lose some of our ability to think logically and quickly. This ability is called cognition (kog-NI-shun). When we lose some of this ability we are said to have cognitive impairment (KOG-ni-tiv im-PAYR-ment). Cognitive impairment affects concentration and memory. Elderly clients may lose their memories of recent events, which can be frustrating for them. You can help by encouraging them to make lists of things to remember and writing down names and phone numbers.

Other normal changes of aging in the brain include slower reaction time, difficulty finding or using the right words, and sleeping less and being more wakeful at night.

Dementia is a more serious loss of mental abilities such as thinking, remembering, reasoning, and communicating. These losses make it difficult to perform ADLs such as eating, bathing, dressing, and toileting. Dementia is not a normal part of aging.

The following are some of the causes of dementia:
- Alzheimer's disease

- Multi-infarct dementia or vascular dementia (a series of strokes that damage the brain)
- Lewy Body disease (also called Lewy Body Dementia)
- Parkinson's disease
- Huntington's disease

Alzheimer's Disease

Alzheimer's disease is a progressive, degenerative, irreversible disease. It causes tangled nerve fibers and protein deposits to form in the brain, eventually causing dementia. Progressive and degenerative mean the disease gets worse, causing greater and greater loss of health and abilities. Irreversible means the disease cannot be cured. Thus, clients with Alzheimer's disease will never recover. They will need more care as the disease progresses.

Alzheimer's disease generally begins with forgetfulness and confusion. It progresses to complete loss of all ability to care for oneself. Each person with Alzheimer's will show different symptoms at different times. For example, one person with Alzheimer's may be able to read, but not able to use the phone or remember her own address. Another person may have lost the ability to read, but may still be able to do simple math. Skills a person has used constantly over a long lifetime are usually kept longer.

Encourage clients with Alzheimer's disease to perform ADLs and keep their minds and bodies as active as possible. Working, socializing, reading, problem solving, and exercising should all be encouraged. Having clients with Alzheimer's do as much as possible for themselves may even help slow the progression of the disease. Look for tasks that are challenging but not frustrating. Help your clients succeed in performing them.

The following attitudes will help you give the best possible care to your clients with Alzheimer's disease:

- Do not take their behavior personally.
- Put yourself in their shoes.
- Treat clients with Alzheimer's disease with dignity and respect, as you would want to be treated.
- Work with the symptoms and behaviors you see.
- Work as a team.

- Take care of yourself.

- Work with family members.

- Remember the goals of the client care plan.

GUIDELINES: COMMUNICATING WITH CLIENTS WHO HAVE ALZHEIMER'S DISEASE

- Speak in a low, calm voice, in a room with little background noise and distraction.

- Repeat yourself, using the same words and phrases as often as needed.

- Use pictures or gestures to communicate.

- Break complex tasks into simple tasks.

Use the same procedures for personal care and ADLs for clients with Alzheimer's disease as you would with other clients. However, there are some guidelines to keep in mind when assisting these clients. Three general principles will help you give your clients the best care:

1 Develop a routine and stick to it. Being consistent is very important when working with clients who are confused and easily upset.

2 Promote self care. Help your clients to care for themselves as much as possible. This will help them cope with this difficult disease.

3 Take good care of yourself, both mentally and physically. This will help you give the best care.

GUIDELINES: CARING FOR CLIENTS WITH ALZHEIMER'S DISEASE

- Ensure safety by using non-slip mats, tub seats, and hand-holds.

- Schedule bathing when the client is least agitated. Be organized so the bath can be quick.

- Always use the same steps, explaining in the same way every time.

- Assist with grooming. Help the people in your care feel attractive and dignified.

- Lay out clothes in the order in which they should be put on. Choose clothes that are simple to put on.

- Set up a regular schedule for toileting and follow it. Never withhold or discourage fluids because a person is incontinent.

- Mark the restroom with a sign as a reminder to use it and where it is.

- Prevent infections. Follow proper procedures for food preparation and storage, household management, and Standard Precautions.

- Maintain a daily exercise routine.

- Maintain the best nutrition. Schedule meals at the same time each day. Serve familiar foods. Try smaller, more frequent meals if person is restless. Finger foods can allow eating while moving around. Keep bite-sized snacks nearby, especially favorites.

- Encourage fluids.

- Maintain self-esteem by encouraging independence in ADLs.

- Share in enjoyable activities, looking at pictures, talking, and reminiscing.

- Reward positive and independent behavior with smiles, hugs, warm touches, and thank yous.

Below are some common difficult behaviors that you may face when working with Alzheimer's clients:

- **Agitation.** Try to eliminate triggers. Keep routine constant. Avoid frustration. Help client focus on a soothing, familiar activity, such as sorting things or looking at pictures. Remain calm and use a low, soothing voice to speak to and reassure the client. An arm around the shoulder, patting, or stroking may be soothing for some clients.

- **Pacing and Wandering.** A client who walks back and forth in the same area is pacing. A client who walks aimlessly around the house or neighborhood is wandering. Pacing and wandering may be caused by restlessness, hunger, disorientation, need for toileting, constipation, pain, forgetting how or where to sit down, too much daytime napping or the need for exercise. Eliminate causes when you can. Let clients pace and wander in a safe and secure (locked) area where you can watch them. Suggest another activity, such as going for a walk.

- **Hallucinations or Delusions.** A client who sees things that are not there is having hallucinations. A client who believes things that are not true is having delusions. Ignore harmless hallucinations and delusions. Reassure a client who seems agitated or worried. Do not argue with a client who is imagining things. Be calm and reassure client that you are there to help.

- **Sundowning.** When a person becomes restless and agitated in the late afternoon, evening, or night, it is called sundowning. Remove triggers. Provide snacks or encourage rest. Avoid stressful situations during this time. Limit activities, appointments, trips, and visits. Play soft music. Set a bedtime routine and keep it. Recognize when sundowning occurs and plan a calming activity just before. Eliminate caffeine from the diet. Give a soothing back massage. Distract the client with a simple, calm activity like looking at a magazine. Maintain a daily exercise routine.

- **Perseveration or Repetitive Phrasing.** A client who repeats a word, phrase, question, or activity over and over is perseverating (per-SEV-er-ayt-ing). Respond to perseveration with patience. Do not try to silence or stop the client. Answer questions each time they are asked, using the same words each time.

- **Violent Behavior.** A client who attacks, hits, or threatens someone is violent. Violence may be triggered by many situations, including frustration, overstimulation, or a change in routine, environment, or caregiver. Look for ways to avoid these triggers.

The following are appropriate responses to violent clients:

- Block blows but never hit back.

- Step out of reach.

- Call for help if needed.

- Do not leave client in the home alone.

- Try to eliminate triggers.

- Use techniques to calm client as you would for agitation or sundowning.

Although Alzheimer's cannot be cured, there are techniques that can improve the quality of life for clients with Alzheimer's.

Reality orientation involves the use of calendars, clocks, signs, and lists to help clients remember who and where they are. It useful in the early stages of Alzheimer's when clients are confused but not totally disoriented. In later stages, reality orientation may only frustrate clients.

Validation therapy means letting clients believe they live in the past or in imaginary circumstances. Validating means giving value to or approving. Make no attempt to reorient clients to actual circumstances. Explore clients' beliefs. Do not argue with them. It is useful in cases of moderate to severe disorientation.

Reminiscence therapy is encouraging clients to remember and talk about the past. Explore memories by asking about details. Focus on a time of life that was more pleasant. Work through feelings about a difficult time in the past. It is useful in many stages of Alzheimer's, but especially with moderate to severe confusion.

Activity therapy uses activities clients enjoy to prevent boredom and frustration. These activities also promote self-esteem. Help clients to take walks, do puzzles, listen to music, cook, read, or do other activities they enjoy. It is useful throughout most stages of Alzheimer's.

Chronic Obstructive Pulmonary Disease (COPD)

Chronic obstructive pulmonary disease, or COPD, is a chronic disease. This means the client may live for years with it but never be cured. Clients with COPD have difficulty breathing, especially in getting air out of the lungs. There are four different chronic lung diseases that are categorized under COPD. They are:

- Chronic bronchitis
- Pulmonary emphysema
- Asthma
- Chronic bronchiectasis

Over time, a client with any of these lung disorders becomes chronically ill and weakened. There is a high risk for acute lung infections, such as pneumonia. When the lungs and brain do not get enough oxygen, all body systems are affected. Clients may live with a constant fear of not being able to breathe. This can cause them to sit upright in an attempt to improve their ability to expand the lungs. These clients can have poor appetites. They usually do not get enough sleep. All of this can add to their feelings of weakness and poor health. They may feel they have lost control of their bodies, and particularly with breathing. They may fear suffocation.

Clients with COPD may experience the following symptoms:

- chronic cough or wheeze
- difficulty breathing, especially with inhaling and exhaling deeply
- shortness of breath, especially during physical exertion
- pale or cyanotic (blue) skin or reddish-purple skin
- mental confusion
- general state of weakness
- difficulty completing meals due to shortness of breath
- fear and anxiety

GUIDELINES: CARING FOR CLIENTS WITH COPD

- Colds or viruses can make clients very ill quickly. Always observe and report signs of symptoms getting worse.

- Help clients sit upright or lean forward. Offer pillows to support them.

- Offer plenty of fluids and small, frequent meals.

- Encourage a well-balanced diet.

- Keep oxygen supply available as ordered.

- Being unable to breathe or fearing suffocation can be very frightening. Be calm and supportive.

- Use good infection control, especially with handwashing by the client and the disposal of used tissues.

- Encourage as much independence with ADLs as possible.

- Remind clients to avoid situations where they may be exposed to infections, especially colds and the flu.

- Teach pursed-lip breathing. Pursed-lip breathing is placing the lips as if in a kiss and taking controlled breaths.

- Encourage clients to save energy for important daily tasks. Encourage clients to rest during tasks.

COPD: OBSERVING AND REPORTING

- temperature over 101°F

- changes in breathing patterns, including shortness of breath

- changes in color or consistency of lung secretions

- changes in mental state or personality

- refusal to take medications as ordered

- excessive weight loss

- increasing dependence upon caregivers and family

Hip/Knee Replacement

Total hip replacement is surgery that replaces the head of the long bone of the leg (femur) where it joins the hip. This may be performed for any of the following reasons:

- Fractured hip due to an injury or fall which does not heal properly

- Weakened hip due to aging

- Hip that is painful and stiff because the joint is weak and the bones are no longer strong enough to bear the weight of the person

The surgery is done through an incision at the hip. An artificial ball and socket joint replaces the hip. After the surgery, the client cannot stand on that leg while the area heals. A physical therapist will help with rehabilitation. The goals of care include slowly strengthening the hip muscles and getting the client walking on that leg.

Be familiar with the care plan. It will state when the client may begin putting weight on the leg. It will also tell how much the client is able to do. It is important to help with personal care and using assistive devices, such as walkers or canes.

GUIDELINES: CARING FOR CLIENTS RECOVERING FROM HIP REPLACEMENTS

- Keep often-used items, such as medications, telephone, tissues, call signals, and water within easy reach. Avoid placing items in high places.

- Dress starting with the affected side first.

- Never rush the client. Use praise and encouragement often. Do this even for small accomplishments.

- Have the client sit to do tasks to save his or her energy.

- Follow the care plan exactly, even if the client wants to do more than is ordered.

- Never perform range of motion exercises on a leg on the side of a hip replacement unless directed by your supervisor.

- Caution the client not to cross legs or turn toes inward. The hip cannot be bent more than 90 degrees. The hip cannot be turned inward. Sometimes an order will limit the operated hip from being turned outward.

HIP REPLACEMENT: OBSERVING AND REPORTING

- incision is red, draining, or warm to touch

- an increase in pain

- abnormal vital signs, especially elevated temperature

- if the client is unable to use equipment properly and safely

- if the client is not following doctor's orders for activity and exercise

- any problems with appetite

- increasing strength and improving ability to walk

Total knee replacement is the surgical insertion of a prosthetic knee. A prosthesis is an artificial body part. This is performed to relieve severe pain and to restore motion to a knee damaged by injury or arthritis. It is also done to help stabilize a knee that buckles or gives out repeatedly. Care is similar to that for a hip replacement. However, the recovery time is much shorter. These clients have more ability to care for themselves. Therefore, they are not seen in home care as often as clients with hip replacements.

VI
Home Management and Nutrition

17. The Client's Environment

Housekeeping

Providing a safe, clean, and orderly environment has always been an essential part of home health care. Clients feel better physically and psychologically and recover more quickly when their homes and families receive care and support. Infection and accidents are prevented. You will be a role model for your clients and their families by demonstrating the following two qualities:

1 Efficiency and Planning. It takes efficiency and planning as well as knowledge and skills to manage a household.

2 Sensitivity. As with all your duties, you must respect the customs, beliefs, and feelings of your clients and their families.

Your assignments will vary. They may include simple cleaning and organizing of the client's room or general cleaning throughout the house. Some clients require management of all household functions, including finances. You may be required to dust, straighten up, vacuum, sweep, wash dishes, clean the bathroom and kitchen, and do laundry. Your assignments will outline the specific duties to be performed.

Most assignments require HHAs to perform light housekeeping. This usually involves dusting, straightening, vacuuming or sweeping floors, cleaning bathrooms and the kitchen, and disposing of trash.

GUIDELINES: HOUSEKEEPING

- Invite family participation. Depending on their abilities and availability, clients and family members may be asked to participate in housekeeping tasks.

- Invite family and client input when you determine the tasks that need to be done and the methods to be used.

- Use cleaning materials and methods that are acceptable to and approved by clients and their families.

- Any efforts you make toward improving the home environment should coincide with the client's choices, lifestyle, and values.

- Be organized when performing tasks. Write out detailed daily and weekly schedules. Seek feedback from your supervisor and the client and family.

- Build some flexibility in the schedule to allow for changes in the client's condition, needs, appointments, or social activities.

- Organize cleaning materials and equipment by placing them in one closet. Do not leave cleaning equipment around the house.

- Familiarize yourself with the household's cleaning materials and equipment. Read the labels and instruction booklets.

- Maintain a safe environment as well as a clean and healthy one. Do not wax floors if your client is unsteady. Mop up spills immediately.

- Use housekeeping procedures and methods that promote good health.

- Observe the home for signs of infestation by roaches, rats, mice, lice, and fleas. Report to your supervisor if you note signs of infestation.

- Use good body mechanics while performing home maintenance activities to prevent injury.

- Clean up and straighten up after every activity. Spills that have dried are difficult to remove later.

- Carry paper and a small pencil to make note of items that must be purchased or replaced. Maintain a shopping list on a bulletin board, refrigerator door, or other convenient location. Encourage family members to use the list.

- Use your time wisely and efficiently. For example, prepare food while a load of wash is being done.

All cleaning products must be used properly. Cleaning products are chemicals, which can be irritating and can even cause burns. Some chemicals are poisonous when swallowed.

GUIDELINES: USING HOUSEHOLD CLEANING PRODUCTS

- Read and follow the directions on the label of every product you use. Cleaning products can harm the materials and surfaces you are trying to clean.

- Do not mix cleaning products. The fumes are toxic and can be fatal.

- Open windows when cleaning to provide fresh air. Some cleaning products may have fumes that are unpleasant or even harmful if you are exposed to them for a long time.

- Do not leave cleaning products on surfaces longer than the recommended time. Do not scrub too hard on some surfaces.

Not all housekeeping tasks must be performed daily. Some tasks may be done weekly. Others only need to be done once a month or seasonally. Space out the special tasks. Do each cleaning job properly and efficiently. Do not take a lot of steps and do not reach, bend, and stoop unnecessarily. Experiment a little to find the most comfortable and effective way to do a job. Cleaning can be done when your client is resting, sleeping, or doing another activity. Care of the client is your primary responsibility. However, do not neglect housekeeping.

GUIDELINES: STRAIGHTENING AND CLEANING LIVING AREAS

- Clear up clutter and put objects in their correct places.

- Pick up newspapers, magazines, and toys as needed.

- Empty wastebaskets and ashtrays daily.

- Make the beds each day.

- Keep essential and frequently-used items, such as eyeglasses, tissues, wastebaskets, newspapers, magazines, and books, within reach.

- Dust once a week or when necessary. If your client has allergies, you may need to dust daily.

- Vacuum floors and rugs once a week or more often if indicated. If the home does not have a vacuum, use a broom to sweep the floors and rugs. Take care not to raise much dust.

- Floors covered with vinyl, ceramic tile, and linoleum may be washed. Wood floors may not. Check with the client or family members before you begin. After removing loose dirt or crumbs with a vacuum or broom, wash floors with a cloth or mop dipped in warm sudsy water. Dry the floor after you have washed it or close off the area for the time it takes for the floor to dry.

Handling food on contaminated surfaces, improper dishwashing, and contaminated food storage areas may transmit many diseases. Roaches, rats, and mice may cause disease by contaminating food with their saliva or through their droppings. Pest control is vital to health and cleanliness. Always report pest control problems to your supervisor.

GUIDELINES: CLEANING THE KITCHEN

- Clean the kitchen after every use. Ask family members to do the same. Do not wait until the end of the day to clean up. Daily kitchen cleaning tasks include washing dishes, wiping surfaces, taking out garbage, and storing leftover food.

- Weekly tasks include cleaning the refrigerator and washing the floor. Cleaning cabinets, drawers, and other storage areas is usually done a few times a year.

- Wash dishes in hot soapy water using liquid dish detergent. Rinse them in hot water. When working with clients who have an infectious disease or a cold, use boiling water for rinsing and add a tablespoon of chlorine bleach to the soapy water. The combination of heat and chlorine will kill pathogens, or harmful microorganisms.

- Wash glasses and cups first, then silverware, plates, and bowls. Pots and pans are washed last. Rinse with hot water and dry on a rack. Air drying dishes is more sanitary than drying them with a dish towel.

- If the house has a dishwasher, learn how to correctly load and start it. Dishwashers save time. They can also sterilize dishes due to the high temperatures used in washing and drying.

- Do not wash the following items in the dishwasher: electrical appliances, certain plastic materials, wooden pieces or utensils, hand-painted or antique dishes, delicate china, crystal, cast iron, most pots and pans, and sharp or carbon steel knives.

- Use only a dishwasher detergent in the dishwasher. Fill the well with only the amount recommended on the label.

- The refrigerator should be totally cleaned once a week. However, you should wipe it out more frequently. To defrost a freezer, turn the dial to the "off" position. Read the directions on the freezer.

- Clean countertops, tables, and the stove each time they are used. Clean cabinet and drawer fronts once a week. If a cutting board or other surface has been used to cut fresh meat, scrub the surface thoroughly with soap and bleach. Rinse well.

- An all-purpose cleaner may be needed to remove grease and cooked foods that have spilled or splashed on surfaces. Clean the sink with a cleanser such as scouring powder or cream.

- Never place food on soiled work or storage areas or in unclean containers. Keep food covered. Close lids of cartons and cover food storage containers to prevent contamination or infestation by insects and rodents. Place leftovers in covered containers and store them in the refrigerator immediately. Use them within two to three days.

- Vacuum, sweep, or dry mop the floor daily. Damp mop uncarpeted floors at least once a week, using hot water and a floor cleaner. Rinse the floor if recommended on the label. Dry the floor or close off the area until the floor dries.

- Dispose of garbage daily. To prevent odor and discourage insects and rodents, rinse out tin cans and bottles before placing them in the garbage pail or recycling bin. Learn and follow the recycling procedures for your client's community. Periodically wash wastebaskets and trash cans with hot, soapy water.

- Store all cleaning materials away from food, food preparation utensils, and food preparation areas. Keep them out of reach of children and confused clients.

A clean, organized, and odor-free bathroom is an important part of improving a family's hygiene and safety. Because it is moist and warm, the bathroom is a reservoir for the growth of microorganisms, mold, and mildew.

Teach all family members basic bathroom hygiene:

- flush the toilet each time it is used
- clean toothbrushes and toothbrush holders often
- scrub the tub and shower after use
- remove hair from drain strainers
- hang up all used towels to dry
- put away toiletries after use
- rinse the sink after brushing teeth, shaving, and washing
- place soiled towels in the laundry hamper after they are dry

The bathroom is the location of many home accidents. Make sure that all bathroom rugs are non-skid. Wipe up puddles of water immediately. If grab bars are not present and your client has difficulty moving about in the bathroom safely, report this to your supervisor.

Cleaning a bathroom

Equipment: disinfectant (a cleaning product that kills germs), scouring powder or scouring cream with bleach, sponge, toilet brush, glass cleaner, paper towels, disposable or rubber gloves

1 Put on gloves.

2 Using the disinfectant and sponge, wipe all surfaces and rinse as needed. Be sure to clean the sides, walls, and curtain or door of the shower or tub; the towel racks; holders for toilet

paper, toothbrushes, and soap; and window sills.

3   Rinse sponge well or use a different sponge to wipe the outside of toilet bowl, seat, and lid. As a general cleaning rule, start with the cleanest surface first, then move to dirtier areas.

4   Use a different sponge to clean the bathtub, shower stall, and sink. Use scouring powder or cream for tile and porcelain, and disinfectant or all-purpose cleaner on other surfaces. Remember that scouring powder can scratch. Check with the client or a family member before using it. Be sure to scrub the sides, edges, and bottoms of all these areas. Clean faucets and scrub around their bases.

5   Scrub the inside of the toilet bowl with a brush and scouring powder containing bleach. Be sure to scrub under the rim. If you use a second, stronger toilet cleaner, flush the first cleaning product down the drain first to avoid possible chemical reactions. Wash the toilet brush with a disinfectant solution and store it in a plastic bag or holder after letting it air dry.

6   Vacuum or dry mop the floor first, then wash if the floor is tile or linoleum. Use an all-purpose floor cleaner in hot water. Wash the floor with a cloth or mop, taking special care to clean the area at the base of the toilet and sink. Do not leave the floor wet. Dry it carefully to avoid accidents.

7   Clean the mirror and any glass or chrome surfaces using glass cleaner and paper towels or clean rags.

8   Place dry, soiled towels in the laundry hamper. Empty the waste can into a plastic or paper garbage bag and dispose of it. Replace toilet tissue and facial tissue when needed. Open the bathroom window for a short time, if possible, to air the room out. Once a week, wash out the waste can and laundry hamper, and launder the bath mats and rugs.

9   Store supplies.

10 Remove and dispose of or store gloves.

11 Wash your hands.

12 Document the cleaning.

GUIDELINES: CLEANING AND ORGANIZING STORAGE AREAS

- Every item in the home should have a storage place that is convenient for use. That means storage places should be as close as possible to where items are used. For example, bath towels should be stored in or near the bathroom. Items that are used together should be stored near each other. Arrange food on shelves according to category. Store dangerous materials out of reach of children and confused adults.

- Some storage areas only need to be cleaned occasionally. Remove the stored items. Wipe the shelves and drawers with a damp cloth and cleaner. Clean food storage areas more often.

- Do not change the client's or the family's storage arrangements without talking to them. If you think changes are needed, discuss your ideas with the family.

Several types of cleaning solutions can be prepared from common household items when supplies are not available or when the family budget is restricted.

- Baking soda can be used instead of scouring powder. Baking soda can also be diluted with warm water to make a solution that will eliminate odors when used to clean surfaces.

- White vinegar can be used to remove lime or other mineral deposits on sinks, toilets, or chrome fixtures. White vinegar diluted with water can be used instead of glass cleaner. Mix solution using one part white vinegar to three parts water (1:3).

- Household bleach, diluted with four parts water, makes a strong disinfectant solution to clean bathroom surfaces. Diluted with ten parts water and stored in a spray bottle, bleach makes a milder disinfectant to use on kitchen counters.

Most housecleaning tasks should be done either immediately, daily, weekly, monthly, or less often. Take into account the care plan, your assigned tasks, how much help is needed, and how much time you have in a particular home to prepare a cleaning schedule. You may not always stick to the schedule exactly. However, it will guide your work and help you get essential cleaning done. Establishing a schedule for cleaning can also help the family keep a housekeeping routine after your assignment has ended.

You must follow Standard Precautions with every client. This is true because you cannot know when infection is present. Special infection control precautions in housecleaning include:

- Use disinfectant when cleaning countertops and surfaces in the kitchen and bathroom.

- Clean the client's bathroom daily. Have other family members use a different bathroom if possible.

- Use separate dishes and utensils for the infected client. In some cases, disposable dishes and utensils will be ordered.

- Wash dishes and utensils in the dishwasher or wash dishes in hot soapy water with bleach. Rinse in boiling water, and allow to air dry.

- Disinfect any surfaces that contact body fluids, such as bedpans, urinals and toilets.

- Frequently remove trash containing used tissues.

- Keep any specimens of urine, stool, or sputum in double bags and away from food and food preparation areas.

Laundry

You may be expected to do hand or machine washing as part of an assignment. Clean clothes, bed linens, and towels are important for hygiene and comfort. In the home, the family and the aide must see that clean clothes and linen are always available for the client.

Laundry Products and Equipment. To do the laundry you will need laundry detergent, a washing machine or a basin for hand washing clothes, and a dryer or a clothesline and pins. The instructions for using washing machines are usually located on the inside of the washing machine lid.

In general, you will use all-purpose detergent. Some delicate fabrics, underwear, or stockings may require a special detergent. Some clients may prefer a non-detergent soap for use on baby clothes and diapers. Bleach, color brighteners, stain removers, and fabric softeners may also be used. Ask the client and family members about their preferences for laundry products.

Pretreating. Pretreating means giving special treatment to items that have heavy soil, spots, and stains before washing them. Spots and stains should be treated immediately. The sooner they are treated, the easier they are to remove. Some oily stains harden with age and cannot be removed.

Bleach. Bleach is used with detergent. However, bleach cannot be used on all fabrics. Be familiar with the type of bleach and the fabric that is being washed. Three types of bleach are used in laundry: liquid chlorine, powdered chlorine, and oxygen or all-fabric. Each type of bleach should be used with caution. Read the instructions on the container carefully. Liquid chlorine bleaches are excellent stain removers. They whiten clothing. However, they can be very damaging to fabric. Bleach should always be diluted in water. Fill the washer, then add liquid bleach. Stir the water before adding clothing. Never use liquid chlorine bleach on silk, spandex, wool, or any item that contains these fibers. Be careful not to spray or splash liquid chlorine bleach. It will remove color or damage fabric.

Water Temperature. Read the washing instructions for all materials and garments. Warm water is the safest temperature for most garments. However, some must be washed in cold to prevent shrinking or colors fading. Hot water is generally used for towels, bed linens, and white or colorfast cottons. Warm is usually used for permanent press, knit, synthetic, sheer, lace, acetate, fabric blends, washable rayons, and plastic. Cold water is used for brightly-colored fabrics or fabrics that are not colorfast.

Washing Action or Cycle. Use the normal setting on the washer for cottons, linens, rayons, sturdy permanent press, knits, synthetics, blends, and most other items. Set the washer on the slow or gentle setting for washable woolens, old quilts, curtains, and delicate or fragile items.

Drying Clothes. Settings on the dryer vary according to the model. Most dryers have a permanent press setting and a delicate setting. The more delicate a fabric, the lower the drying temperature and the shorter the time in the dryer. Heavy items such as towels need higher temperature settings and a longer time in the dryer. Clean the lint filter each time you use the dryer. If your client does not have a clothes dryer, hang clothes on a clothesline using clothespins.

Folding. To reduce the amount of wrinkling, remove all clothes from the dryer immediately. Fold them neatly or place them on hangers. Set aside those that need to be ironed. Return other items to their drawers.

Ironing. Before you begin to iron, check the label of the item for the recommended temperature. If the label does not recommend a particular setting or the fabric is a blend, use the lowest temperature on the iron. Take special care with pile fabrics, such as velvets and corduroy. Use a pressing cloth to protect the fabric and to prevent them from becoming shiny.

Maintaining Clothing. You may need to do basic mending or sewing occasionally. This is especially true if you are taking care of a family, an older person with impaired vision, or people who may not have the time or the ability to keep clothing and linens repaired. Some clients who can do their own mending may just need you to thread the needle.

When a client has a known infectious disease, you must take special precautions when handling laundry:

- Keep client's laundry separate from that of other family members.
- Handle dirty laundry as little as possible. Sort it and put it in plastic bags in the client's room or bathroom. Take it immediately to the laundry area. Keep laundry off the floor.

- Wear gloves and hold laundry away from your clothes and body when you are handling it.

- Use liquid bleach when fabrics allow.

- Use agency-approved disinfectants in all loads.

- Use hot water.

Doing the laundry

1 Sort clothes carefully. Make separate piles of whites, colors, and bright colors. Check clothing labels for special washing instructions. Do not wash anything labeled "Dry Clean Only." If hand-washing is recommended, do not wash in the machine.

2 As you sort laundry, check pockets and remove tissues, money, pens, and other items. Remove belts with buckles, trims, and nonwashable ornaments. Close zippers, buttons, and other fasteners. Check garments for stains and areas of heavy soil. If appropriate, mend or repair any holes, snags, rips, tears, pulled seams, and weak spots in garments and other items.

3 Pretreat spots and stains before washing. A small amount of liquid detergent or dry detergent dissolved in water can be worked in

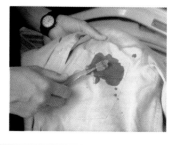

with an old toothbrush. Pretreat or soak clothing as soon as possible for best results. If you know something is spotted, do not let it sit in the laundry hamper all week until you do the laundry.

4 Use the correct water temperature: hot for whites, warm for colors, cold for bright colors.

5 Use the appropriate laundry product(s). Follow the washing instructions on the container.

6 Follow written instructions or client or family instructions for using the washer. Use the correct washing cycle for the load you are laundering.

7 Dry clothes completely either in a dryer or on a clothesline. If using an automatic dryer, follow the drying instructions on clothing labels. Some fabrics require cooler temperatures.

8 Hand-wash items in warm or cool water, depending on the fabric and instructions. Use a mild detergent or special handwashing liquid. Line dry or lay flat on towels to preserve the shape of the garment.

9 Fold or hang clean laundry and sort into categories. Store in drawers or closets.

In some assignments, you will be asked to teach housekeeping skills to family members. This prepares them to take over housekeeping and care when home care is discontinued. By teaching household management skills, you can help families meet their daily needs and become more self-reliant.

Bedmaking

When clients spend much or all of their time in bed, careful bedmaking is essential to their comfort, cleanliness, and health. Linens should always be changed after personal care procedures such as sponge baths, or any time bedding or sheets are damp, soiled, or in need of straightening. The following are three reasons why it is important that clients' bed linens be changed frequently:

1 Sheets that are damp, wrinkled, or bunched up under a client are uncomfortable. They may prevent the client from resting or sleeping well.

2 Microorganisms thrive in moist, warm environments. Bedding that is damp or unclean encourages infection and disease.

3 Clients who spend long hours in bed are at risk for pressure sores. Sheets that do not lie flat under the client's body increase the risk of pressure sores because they cut off circulation.

If a client cannot get out of bed, you must change the linens with the client in bed. When making the bed, be careful to use a wide stance with knees bent. Avoid bending from the waist, especially when tucking sheets or blankets under the mattress. Mattresses can be heavy, so remember to bend your knees to avoid injury. It is easier to make an unoccupied bed than one with a client in it. If the client can be moved temporarily to a chair or other comfortable spot, your job will be easier.

Making an occupied bed

Equipment: clean linen: mattress pad, fitted or flat bottom sheet, waterproof bed protector if needed, cotton draw sheet, flat top sheet, blanket(s), pillowcase(s), gloves (if you are going to be touching linens soiled with body fluids), laundry hamper or basket

1 Wash your hands.

2 Explain the procedure to the client. Speak clearly, slowly, and directly. Maintain face-to-face contact whenever possible.

3 Provide privacy if the client desires it.

4 Place clean linen on clean surface within reach (e.g., bedside stand or chair).

5 If the bed is adjustable, adjust bed to a safe working level, usually waist high. If the bed is movable, lock bed wheels. Lower head of bed.

6 Put on gloves if linens are soiled with body fluids.

7 Loosen top linen from the end of the bed or working side. Cover the client with a cotton bath blanket or the loosened top sheet on the bed.

8 You will make the bed one side at a time. Raise side rail on far side of bed. This protects the client from falling out of the bed while you are making it. After raising the side rail, ask the client to turn

onto side, moving away from you towards raised side rail. If the client cannot roll to the side without assistance, assist him or her to turn onto his or her side, moving away from you toward raised side rail.

9   On working side, with the client's back to you, loosen the bottom soiled linen, mattress pad, and protector if present.

10 Roll bottom soiled linen toward client, tucking it snugly against the client's back.

11 Place and tuck in clean bottom linen. Finish with bottom sheet free of wrinkles. If you are using a flat bottom sheet, leave enough overlap on each end to tuck under the mattress. If the sheet is only long enough to tuck in at one end, tuck it in securely at the top of the bed. Make hospital corners to keep bottom sheet wrinkle-free.

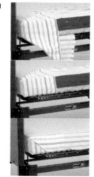

12 Smooth the bottom sheet out toward the client. Be sure there are no wrinkles in the mattress pad. Roll the extra material toward the client. Tuck it under the client's body.

13 If using a waterproof pad, unfold it and center it on the bed. Tuck the side near you under the mattress. Smooth it out toward the client. Tuck as you did with the sheet.

14 If using a draw sheet, place it on the bed. Tuck in on your side, smooth, and tuck as you did with the other bedding.

15 Assist client to turn onto clean bottom sheet. Protect the client from any soiled matter on the old linens. Raise side rail nearest you.

16 Move to other side of the bed and lower the side rail.

17 Turn the client away from you toward side rail.

18 Loosen the soiled linen. Look for personal items. Roll linen from head to the foot of bed. Avoid contact with your skin or clothes. Place it in a hamper or basket. Never put it on the floor or furniture. Never shake it. Soiled bed linens are full of microorganisms that should not be spread to other parts of the room.

19 Pull and tuck in clean bottom linen just like the other side. Finish with bottom sheet free of wrinkles.

20 Ask client to turn onto his or her back. Keep client covered and comfortable, with a pillow under the head. Raise side rail.

21 Unfold the top sheet and place it over the client. Ask the client to hold the top sheet. Slip the blanket or old sheet out from underneath. Put it in the laundry hamper.

22 Place a blanket over the top sheet, matching the top edges. Tuck the bottom edges of top sheet and blanket under the bottom of the mattress. Make hospital corners on each side. Loosen the top linens over the client's feet. This prevents pressure on the feet. At the top of the bed, fold the top sheet over the blanket about six inches.

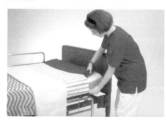

23 Remove the pillow. Do not hold it near your face. Remove the soiled pillowcase by turning it inside out. Place it in the laundry hamper.

24 With one hand, grasp the clean pillowcase at the closed end. Turn it inside out over your arm. Next, using the same hand that has the pillowcase over it, grasp one narrow edge of the pillow. Pull the pillowcase over it with your free hand. Do the same for any other pillows. Place them under your client's head or as client desires.

25 If you raised an adjustable bed, be sure to return it to its lowest position. Put any signaling device within the client's reach.

26 Carry laundry hamper to laundry area. Remove gloves if worn.

27 Wash your hands.

28 Document the procedure and any observations.

Making an unoccupied bed

Equipment: clean linen: mattress pad, fitted or flat bottom sheet, waterproof bed protector if needed, cotton draw sheet, flat top sheet, blanket(s), pillowcase(s), gloves (if you are going to be touching linens soiled with body fluids), laundry hamper or basket

1 Wash your hands.

2 Place clean linen on clean surface within reach (e.g., bedside stand or chair).

3 If the bed is adjustable, adjust bed to a safe working level, usually waist high. If the bed is movable, lock bed wheels. Put bed in flattest position.

4 Put on gloves if linens are soiled with body fluids.

5 Loosen soiled linen. Roll soiled linen (soiled side inside) from head to foot of bed. Avoid contact with your skin or clothes. Place it in a hamper or basket.

6 Remove gloves. Wash your hands.

7 Remake the bed. Spread mattress pad and bottom sheet and tuck under. Make hospital corners to keep bottom sheet wrinkle-free. Put on mattress protector and draw sheet. Smooth and tuck under sides of bed.

8 Place top sheet and blanket over bed. Center these, tuck under end of bed and make hospital corners. Fold down the top sheet over the blanket about six inches. Fold both top sheet and blanket down so client can easily get into bed. If client will not be returning to bed immediately, leave bedding up.

9 Remove pillows and pillowcases. Remove gloves. Put on clean pillowcases (as described in procedure above). Replace pillows.

10 If you raised an adjustable bed, be sure to return it to its lowest position. Put any signaling device within the client's reach. Carry laundry hamper to laundry area. Remove gloves if worn.

11 Wash your hands.

12 Document the procedure and any observations.

18. Proper Nutrition

Nutrition

Good nutrition is very important. Nutrition is how the body uses food to maintain health. Our bodies need a well-balanced diet containing essential nutrients and plenty of fluids. This helps us grow new cells, maintain normal body function, and have energy for activities. Good nutrition in childhood and early adulthood helps ensure good health later in life. For those who are ill or elderly, a well-balanced diet helps maintain muscle and skin tissues and prevent pressure sores. A good diet promotes the healing of wounds. It also helps us cope with physical and emotional stress.

The Six Basic Nutrients

The body needs the following nutrients for growth and development:

1 **Protein.** Proteins are part of every body cell. They are essential for tissue growth and repair. Proteins are also an alternate supply of energy for the body. Excess proteins are excreted by the kidneys or stored as body fat.

   Sources include fish, seafood, poultry, meat, eggs, milk, cheese, nuts, peas, and dried beans or legumes. Whole grain cereals, pastas, rice, and breads contain some proteins of lower quality. They must be complemented by a small quantity of the more complete proteins. Beans and rice or cereal and milk are examples of complementary proteins.

2 **Carbohydrates**. Carbohydrates supply the fuel for the body's energy needs. They supply extra protein and help the body use fat efficiently. Carbohydrates also provide fiber, which is necessary for bowel elimination.

   Carbohydrates can be divided into two basic types: complex and simple carbohydrates. Complex carbohydrates are found in foods such as bread, cereal, potatoes, rice, pasta, vegetables, and fruits. Simple carbohydrates are found in foods such as sugars, sweets, syrups, and jellies. Simple carbohydrates do not have the same nutritional value as complex carbohydrates do. The only value of simple carbohydrates is as energy for people who eat very little or are malnourished. In others, simple carbohydrates are stored as fat.

3 **Fats.** Fat helps the body store energy. Body fat also provides the body with insulation. It protects body organs. In addition, fats add flavor to food and are important for the absorption of certain vitamins. Excess fat in the diet is stored as fat in the body.

   Examples of fats are butter, margarine, salad dressings, oils, and animal fats found in meats, fowl, and fish. Monounsaturated vegetable fats (including olive oil and canola oil) and polyunsaturated vegetable fats (including corn and safflower oils) are healthier kinds of fats.

Saturated fats, including animal fats like butter, lard, bacon and other fatty meats, are not as healthy. They should be limited in most diets.

4 **Vitamins.** Vitamins are substances the body needs to function. The body cannot produce most vitamins. They can only be obtained from food. Vitamins A, D, E, and K are fat-soluble vitamins. This means they are carried and stored in body fat. Vitamins B and C are water-soluble vitamins that are broken down by water in our bodies. They cannot be stored in the body. They are eliminated in urine and feces.

5 **Minerals.** Minerals form and maintain body functions. They provide energy and regulate processes. Zinc, iron, calcium, and magnesium are examples of minerals. Minerals are found in many foods.

6 **Water.** Because one-half to two-thirds of our body weight is water, we need about 8 glasses, or 64 ounces, of water or other fluids a day. Water is the most essential nutrient for life. Without it, a person can only live a few days. Water assists in the digestion and absorption of food. It helps with the elimination of waste. Through perspiration, water also helps maintain normal body temperature. Maintaining fluid balance in our bodies is necessary for good health.

Most foods contain several nutrients, but no one food contains all the nutrients that are necessary to maintain a healthy body. Therefore, it is important that we eat a daily diet that is well-balanced. There is not one single dietary plan that is right for everyone. People have different nutritional and calorie intake needs depending upon their age, gender, and activity level.

In 1980, the U.S. Department of Agriculture (USDA) developed the Food Guide Pyramid to help promote healthy eating practices. In 2005, in response to new scientific information about nutrition and health and new technology for support tools, MyPyramid was developed. MyPyramid replaces the Food Guide Pyramid. MyPyramid is a personalized version of the Food Guide Pyramid that offers individual plans based on age, gender, and activity level.

The Pyramid is made up of six bands of different widths and colors. Each color represents a food group—orange for grains, green for vegetables, maroon for fruits, yellow for oils, blue for milk, and purple for meat and beans. The different widths indicate that not all groups should make up an equal part of a healthy diet. The orange band, grains, is the widest. This means that grains should make up the highest proportion of the diet. The smaller bands, such as the purple band representing meat and beans, should make up a smaller part of foods eaten. The smallest band, the yellow one, represents oils. Oils contain essential fatty acids. However, this band is not emphasized because the body needs fats and oils in smaller quantities.

The bands of the Pyramid are wide at the bottom and narrow into a point at the top. This is a reminder that there are a great variety of foods that make up each group. Many choices are available to help meet the daily requirements. Foods that are nutrient-dense and low in fat and calories should form the "base" of a healthy diet. They are represented by the wide base of the Pyramid. Foods that are high in fat and sugar and have less nutritional value are at the narrow top. They should be eaten less often.

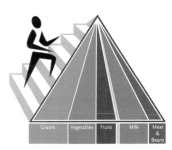

The new Pyramid also emphasizes the importance of physical activity, as represented by the figure climbing the stairs. Physical activity goes hand-in-hand with diet to make up an overall healthy lifestyle. The USDA recommends at least 30 minutes per day of vigorous activity for everyone. Sixty minutes or more is even better.

Grains. The grains group includes all foods made from wheat, rice, oats, cornmeal, and barley. Examples are bread, pasta, oatmeal, breakfast cereals, tortillas and grits. One slice of bread, one cup of ready-to-eat cereal, or ½ cup of cooked rice, pasta, or cooked cereal can be considered a one ounce equivalent from the grains group.

There are two subgroups of grains: whole grains and refined grains. Whole grains contain the entire grain kernel. Refined grains have been milled, a process that removes the bran and germ. This gives grain a finer texture and improves its shelf life but also removes dietary fiber, iron, and many B vitamins. At least half of all grains consumed should be whole grains. Words to look for on food labels to ensure that grains are whole grains are: brown rice, wild rice, bulgur, oatmeal, whole-grain corn, whole oats, whole wheat, and whole rye. Words that do not usually indicate whole grains include multi-grain, stone-ground, 100% wheat, cracked wheat, seven-grain, or bran.

Vegetables. Vegetables. The vegetable group includes all fresh, frozen, canned and dried vegetables and vegetable juices. One cup of raw or cooked vegetables or vegetable juice or two cups of raw leafy greens can be considered as one cup from the vegetable group. There are five sub-groups within the vegetable group. They are organized by nutritional content. These are dark green vegetables, orange vegetables, dry beans and peas, starchy vegetables, and other vegetables. A variety of vegetables from these subgroups should be eaten every day. Dark green vegetables, orange vegetables, and dried beans and peas have the best nutritional content.

Vegetables are low in fat and calories and have no cholesterol (although sauces and seasonings may add fat, calories and cholesterol). They are good sources of dietary fiber, potassium, Vitamin A, Vitamin E, and Vitamin C.

Fruits. The fruit group includes all fresh, frozen, canned and dried fruits and fruit juices. One cup of fruit or 100% fruit juice or ½ cup of dried fruit can be considered as one cup from the fruit group. Most choices should be whole or cut up fruit rather than juice for the additional dietary fiber provided.

Fruits, like vegetables, are naturally low in fat, sodium and calories and have no cholesterol. They are important sources of dietary fiber and many nutrients, including folic acid and Vitamin C.

Milk. The milk group includes all fluid milk products and foods made from milk that retain their calcium content, such as yogurt and cheese. Foods made from milk that have little to no calcium, such as cream cheese, cream, and butter, are not part of the group. Most milk group choices should be fat-free or low-fat. One cup of milk or yogurt, one and a half ounces of natural cheese, or two ounces of processed cheese can be considered as one cup from the milk group.

Foods in the milk group provide nutrients that are vital for the health and maintenance of your body. These nutrients include calcium, potassium, Vitamin D, and protein. Calcium is used for building bones and teeth and in maintaining bone mass. Milk products are the primary source of calcium in American diets.

Meat and Beans. One ounce of lean meat, poultry, or fish, one egg, one tablespoon peanut butter, ¼ cup cooked dry beans, or ½ ounce of nuts or seeds can be considered as one ounce equivalent from the meat and beans group. Dry beans and peas can be included as part of this group or part of the vegetable group. If meat is eaten regularly, they should be included with vegetables. If not, they should be included as part of this group.

Most meat and poultry choices should be lean or low-fat. Diets that are high in saturated fats raise "bad" cholesterol levels in the blood. Some food choices in this group are high in saturated fat. These include fatty cuts of beef, pork, and lamb; regular (75% to 85% lean) ground beef; regular sausages, hot dogs, and bacon; some luncheon meats such as regular bologna and salami; and some poultry such as duck. These foods should be limited to help keep blood cholesterol levels healthy.

Fish, nuts, and seeds contain healthy oils. These foods are a good choice instead of meat or poultry. Some nuts and seeds (flax, walnuts) are excellent sources of essential fatty acids. These acids may reduce the risk of cardiovascular disease. Some (sunflower seeds, almonds, hazelnuts) are good sources of vitamin E.

Oils. Oils include fats from many different plants and from fish that are liquid at room temperature, such as canola, corn, olive, soybean and sunflower oil. Some foods are naturally high in oils, like nuts, olives, some fish, and avocados. Foods that are mainly oil include mayonnaise, certain salad dressings, and soft margarine.

Most of the fats you eat should be polyunsaturated (PUFA) or monounsaturated (MUFA) fats. Oils are the major source of MUFAs and PUFAs in the diet. PUFAs contain some fatty acids that are necessary for health. These are called "essential fatty acids."

Most Americans consume enough oil in the foods they eat, such as nuts, fish, cooking oil, and salad dressings.

Activity. Physical activity and nutrition work together for better health. Being active increases the amount of calories burned. As people age, their metabolism slows. Maintaining energy balance requires moving more and eating less. For health benefits, physical activity should be moderate or vigorous and add up to at least 30 minutes a day.

For more information on MyPyramid, visit www.mypyramid.gov.

Most clients should be encouraged to drink at least eight glasses, or 64 ounces, of water a day. Remember that water is an essential nutrient for life. The sense of thirst often diminishes as people age. Remind your elderly clients to drink fluids often. However, some clients may have an order to restrict fluids (RF) or to force fluids (FF) because of medical conditions. Follow your client's care plan.

Dehydration occurs when a person does not have enough fluid in the body. Dehydration is a serious condition. People can become dehydrated if they do not drink enough or they have diarrhea or are vomiting.

DEHYDRATION: OBSERVING AND REPORTING

Report any of the following immediately:

- if a client drinks less than eight 8-ounce glasses of liquid per day
- if a client needs help drinking from a cup
- if a client has trouble swallowing liquids
- if a client experiences frequent vomiting, diarrhea, or fever
- if client is easily tired or confused

Report if the client has any of the following:

- dry mouth
- cracked lips
- sunken eyes
- dark urine
- strong-smelling urine

GUIDELINES: PREVENTING DEHYDRATION

- Report observations and warning signs to your supervisor immediately.
- Encourage your clients to drink every time you see them.
- Offer fresh water or other fluids often.
- Record fluid intake and output if assigned.
- Ice chips, frozen flavored ice sticks, and gelatin are also forms of liquids. Offer them often. Do not offer ice chips or sticks if a client has a swallowing problem.
- If appropriate, offer sips of liquid between bites of food at meals and snacks.
- Make sure a pitcher and cup are near enough and light enough for a client to lift.
- Offer assistance if a client cannot drink without help. Use adaptive cups as needed.

Fluid overload occurs when the body is unable to handle the amount of fluid consumed. This condition often affects people with heart or kidney disease.

FLUID OVERLOAD: OBSERVING AND REPORTING

- swelling/edema of extremities (ankles, feet, fingers, hands)
- weight gain (daily weight gain of one to two pounds)
- decreased urine output
- shortness of breath
- increased heart rate
- skin that appears tight, smooth, and shiny

Aging and illness can lead to emotional and physical problems that affect the intake of food. For example, people who are lonely or who suffer from illnesses that affect their ability to chew and swallow may have little interest in food.

Unintended weight loss is a serious problem for the elderly. Weight loss can mean that the client has a serious medical condition. It can lead to skin breakdown, which leads to pressure sores. It is very important to report any weight loss you notice, no matter how small.

UNINTENDED WEIGHT LOSS: OBSERVING AND REPORTING

Report any of the following immediately:

- if a client needs help eating or drinking
- if a client eats less than 70% of meals/snacks served
- if client has mouth pain
- if a client has dentures that do not fit properly
- if client has any difficulty chewing or swallowing
- if a client coughs or chokes while eating
- if a client is sad, has crying spells, or withdraws from others
- if a client is confused, wanders, or paces

GUIDELINES: PREVENTING UNINTENDED WEIGHT LOSS

- Report observations and warning signs to your supervisor.
- Encourage clients to eat. Talk about food served in a positive tone of voice and with positive words.
- Honor clients' food likes and dislikes.
- Offer different kinds of foods and beverages.
- Help clients who have trouble feeding themselves.

- Food should look, taste, and smell good. The person may have a poor sense of taste and smell.

- Season foods to clients' preferences.

- Allow enough time for clients to finish eating.

- Notify your supervisor if clients have trouble using utensils.

- Record the meal/snack intake if assigned.

- Provide oral care before and after meals.

- Position clients sitting upright for feeding.

- If a client has had a loss of appetite and/or seems sad, ask about it.

If a client has trouble swallowing, soft foods and thickened liquids will be served. You will learn more about thickened liquids later in this section. A straw or special cup will help make swallowing easier.

Swallowing problems cause a high risk for choking on food or drink. Inhaling food or drink into the lungs is called aspiration. Aspiration can cause pneumonia or death. Notify your supervisor immediately if any problems occur while feeding.

GUIDELINES: PREVENTING ASPIRATION

- Position clients properly when eating. They must sit in a straight, upright position. Do not try to feed clients in a reclining position.

- Offer small pieces of food or small spoons of pureed food.

- Feed clients slowly.

- Place food in the non-paralyzed, or unaffected, side of the mouth.

- Make sure mouth is empty before each bite of food or sip of drink.

- Clients should stay in the upright position for about 30 minutes after eating and drinking.

When a person is completely unable to swallow, he or she may be fed through a tube. A nasogastric tube is inserted into the nose and goes to the stomach. A tube can also be placed through the skin directly into the stomach. This is called a PEG (Percutaneous Endoscopic Gastrostomy) tube. The opening in the stomach and abdomen is called a gas-

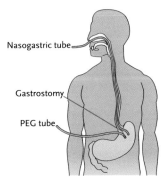

Nasogastric tube

Gastrostomy

PEG tube

trostomy. Tube feedings are used when clients cannot swallow but can digest food.

If a person's digestive system does not function properly, hyperalimentation or total parenteral nutrition (TPN) may be needed. With TPN, a client receives nutrients directly into the bloodstream. It bypasses the digestive system.

Home health aides are not responsible for tube or TPN feedings. You may be assigned to take the person's temperature or assemble supplies for a sterile dressing change. In addition, you should observe, report, and document any observation of changes in the client or problems with the feeding.

When planning meals and cooking for your clients, know their food preferences. Some of these may be listed in the care plan. You will also need to find out more before planning meals. Ask the client or a family member to tell you about food preferences, or suggest some sample menus and ask for reactions. Pay attention to what is eaten when you serve meals. If a client never finishes her chicken, it may mean that she prefers other kinds of meats. Cost may also be a factor in choosing foods. Protein-rich foods are generally the most expensive, but also the most important for the healing process.

The Food and Drug Administration (FDA) requires that all packaged foods contain a standardized nutrition label, called "Nutrition Facts."

The Nutrition Facts label gives you the following information:

- serving size and number of servings per container

- calories per serving and calories from fat per serving

- percentage of daily totals for vitamins and minerals

Regular Frozen Lasagna

Nutrition Facts	
Serving size 1 Package (10.75 oz.)	
Amount Per Serving	
Calories 360	Calories from Fat 120
	% Daily Value
Total Fat 13g	20%
Saturated Fat 7g	35%
Cholesterol 35mg	11%
Sodium 960mg	40%
Total Carbohydrate 40g	14%
Dietary Fiber 6g	23%
Sugars 10g	
Protein 21g	
Calcium	35%
Vitamin A	10%
Vitamin C	10%
Iron	6%

Special Diets

A doctor sometimes places clients who have certain illnesses on special diets. These diets are known as "therapeutic," "modified," or "special" diets. Certain nutrients or fluids may be restricted or eliminated. Some medications may interact with certain foods, which then must be restricted. Clients who do not eat enough may be placed on special supplementary diets. Diets are also prescribed for weight control and food allergies.

You will play an important role in helping clients follow their modified diets. The care plan should specify any special diet the client is on. Never modify a client's diet. Therapeutic diets can only be prescribed by doctors and planned by dietitians. Follow the client's diet plan.

Low-Sodium Diet. People are most familiar with sodium as one of the two ingredients of salt. Salt is the first food to be restricted in a low-sodium diet because it is high in sodium. Foods high in sodium include cured meats: ham, bacon, lunch meat, sausage, salt pork, and hot dogs; salty or smoked fish: herring, salted cod, sardines, anchovies, caviar, smoked salmon or lox; processed cheese; canned and dried soups; vegetables preserved in brine: pickles, sauerkraut, olives, relishes; salted foods: nuts, dips, and spreads; sauces with high concentrations of salt: Worcestershire, barbecue, chili, and soy sauces; ketchup and mustard; canned foods; some cereals; and over-the-counter medications and drugs.

Fluid-Restricted Diet. The amount of fluid taken into the body through food and fluids must equal the amount of fluid that leaves the body through perspiration, stool, urine, and expiration. This is fluid balance. When fluid intake is greater than fluid output, body tissues become swollen with excess fluid. In addition, people with severe heart disease and kidney disease may have difficulty processing large volumes of fluid. To prevent further heart and kidney damage, doctors may restrict a client's fluid intake. For clients on fluid restriction, you will need to measure and document exact amounts of fluid intake. Report excesses to your supervisor. Do not offer additional fluids or foods that count as fluids, such as ice cream, puddings, gelatin, etc. If the client complains of thirst or requests fluids, tell your supervisor.

Low-Protein Diet. People who have kidney disease may also be on low-protein diets. Protein is restricted because it breaks down into compounds that may lead to further kidney damage. The extent of the restrictions depends on the stage of the disease and whether the client is on dialysis.

Low-Fat/Low-Cholesterol Diet. People who have high levels of cholesterol in their blood are at risk for heart attacks and heart disease. People with gallbladder disease, diseases that interfere with fat digestion, and liver disease are also placed on low-fat/low-cholesterol diets. Low-fat/low-cholesterol diets permit skim milk, low-fat cottage cheese, fish, white meat of turkey and chicken, veal, and vegetable fats (especially monounsaturated fats such as olive, canola, and peanut oils). Clients may be advised to limit their diets in these ways:

- Eat lean cuts of meat including lamb, beef, and pork, and eat these only three times a week.

- Limit egg yolks to three or four per week (including eggs used in baking).

- Avoid organ meats, shellfish, fatty meats, cream, butter, lard, meat drippings, coconut and palm oils, and desserts and soups made with whole milk.

- Avoid fried foods and sweets.

People who have gallbladder disease or other digestive problems may be placed on a diet that restricts all fats.

Modified Calorie Diet for Weight Management. Some clients may need to reduce calories to lose weight or prevent additional weight gain. Other clients need to increase calories because of malnutrition, surgery, illness, or fever. Clients with certain conditions need more protein to promote growth and repair of tissue and regulation of body functions.

Dietary Management of Ulcers. Gastric and duodenal (doo-a-DEE-nal) ulcers can be irritated by foods that produce gastric distress or increase levels of acid in the stomach. People who have ulcers usually know the foods that cause them discomfort. Doctors will advise them to avoid these foods as well as the following: alcohol; beverages containing caffeine, such as coffee, tea, and soft drinks; and spicy seasonings such as black pepper, cayenne, and chili pepper. Three meals or more a day are usually advised. If alcohol is allowed, it should be drunk with meals.

Dietary Management of Diabetes. People with diabetes must be very careful about what they eat. Calories and carbohydrates are carefully controlled in the diets of diabetic clients. Protein and fats are also regulated. The foods and the amounts are determined by nutritional and energy needs. See Part V for more information on diabetes.

A dietitian and the client will make up a meal plan together. It will include all the right types and amounts of food for each day. The client uses exchange lists, or lists of similar foods that can substitute for one another, to make up a menu. Using meal plans and exchange lists, a person with diabetes can control his diet while still making food choices.

To keep their blood glucose levels near normal, diabetic clients must eat the right amount of the right type of food at the right time. They must eat all that is served. Encourage them to do so. Do not offer other foods without the doctor's approval. If a client will not eat what is directed, or if you think that he or she is not following the diet, inform your supervisor.

Diets may also be modified in consistency:

Liquid Diets. A liquid diet is made up of foods that are liquid at body temperature. Liquid diets are usually ordered as "clear" or "full." A clear liquid diet includes clear juices, broth, gelatin, and popsicles. A full liquid diet includes clear liquids with the addition of cream soups, milk, and ice cream. A liquid diet is usually ordered for a short time. It may be ordered due to a medical condition or before or after a test or surgery.

Soft Diet. The soft diet is soft in texture. It consists of soft or chopped foods that are easier to chew and swallow. Doctors order this diet for clients who have chewing and swallowing problems due to dental problems or other medical conditions.

Pureed Diet. To puree a food means to chop, blend, or grind it into a thick paste of baby food consistency. The food should be thick enough to hold its form in the mouth. This diet does not need to be chewed. A pureed diet is often used for people who have trouble chewing and/or swallowing more textured foods.

Clients with swallowing problems may be restricted to consuming only thickened liquids. Thickening improves the ability to control fluid in the mouth and throat. A doctor orders the necessary thickness after the client has been evaluated by a speech therapist.

Special products are used for thickening. If thickening is ordered, it must be used with all liquids. You need to know what thickened liquids mean. Do not offer these clients regular liquids. Never offer water to a client who must have thickened liquids. Follow the care plan for each client as ordered.

Three basic thickened consistencies are:

1 **Nectar Thick**: This consistency is thicker than water. It is the thickness of a thick juice, such as a pear nectar or tomato juice. A client can drink this from a cup.

2 **Honey Thick**: This consistency has the thickness of honey. It will pour very slowly. A client will usually use a spoon to consume it.

3 **Pudding Thick**: With this consistency, the liquids have become semi-solid, much like pudding. A spoon should stand up straight in the glass when put into the middle of the drink. A client must consume these liquids with a spoon.

Planning and Shopping

When your meal plan is completed, make your shopping list. On a large sheet of paper, write down categories including produce, meats, canned goods, frozen foods, dairy, and other. Leave space under each category to list the foods you need to buy. Listing items by category will save you time in the grocery store. Go through your plan meal by meal. Write down all of the ingredients you will need for each meal. Remember to include beverages. Check the refrigerator, cabinets, and pantry for ingredients. Many ingredients you need may already be in the home. Keep a shopping list going all the time so family members, clients, and you can write down things you run out of during the week.

GUIDELINES: SHOPPING FOR CLIENTS

- Use coupons. If your client receives a newspaper, scan it for coupons from stores or manufacturers. Clip and use only those coupons for items you have already planned to buy.

- Check store circulars for advertised specials.

- Buy fresh foods that are in season, when they are at peak flavor and inexpensive.

- Buy in quantity. Large amounts or larger sizes are usually more economical, but do not buy more than you can store.

- Shop from your list. Do not be tempted by items that are not on your list.

- Avoid processed, already-mixed, or ready-made foods. They are usually more expensive and less nutritious. When time allows, buy staples.

- Buy a cheaper brand when appearance is not important.

- Read labels to be sure you are getting the kind of product and the quantity you want.

- Estimate the cost per serving before buying. Divide the total cost by the number of servings to determine the cost per serving.

- Consider the amount of waste in bones and fat when buying cheaper cuts of meat.

- Avoid convenience stores. Shopping at large supermarkets or discount stores usually guarantees you will get the best prices.

- Plan ahead. Knowing what you need and buying before you run out will save you money.

When deciding what to buy, keep these four factors in mind:

1 Nutritional value

2 Quality

3 Price

4 Preference

Preparing and Storing

Food-borne illnesses affect up to 100 million people each year. Elderly people are at increased risk partly because they may not see, smell, or taste that food is spoiled. They also may not have the energy to prepare and store food safely. For people who have weakened immune systems because of AIDS or cancer, a food-borne illness can be deadly.

GUIDELINES: SAFE FOOD PREPARATION

- Wash hands frequently. Wash your hands thoroughly before beginning any food preparation. Wash your hands after handling raw meat, poultry, or fish.

- Keep everything clean. Clean and disinfect countertops and other surfaces before, during (as necessary), and after food preparation.

- Handle raw meat, poultry and fish carefully. Use an antibacterial kitchen cleaner or a dilute bleach solution to clean any countertops on which meat juices have spilled. Wrap paper or packaging containing meat juices in plastic and discard immediately.

- Once you have used a knife or cutting board to cut fresh meat, do not use it for anything else until it has been washed in the dishwasher or in very hot, soapy water containing bleach.

- Use plastic cutting boards for raw meat and wooden ones for vegetables and other foods.

- Change dishcloths, sponges and towels frequently. Sponges may be washed in the dishwasher to disinfect them.

- Defrost frozen foods in the refrigerator, not on the countertop. Do not remove meats or dairy products from the refrigerator until just before use.

- Wash fruits and vegetables thoroughly in running water to remove pesticides and bacteria. Cook thoroughly.

- Cook meats, poultry, and fish thoroughly to kill any harmful microorganisms they may contain. Heat leftovers thoroughly. Never leave food out for over two hours. Keep cold foods cold and hot foods hot.

The following basic methods of food preparation will allow you to prepare a variety of healthy meals:

- **Boiling.** Food is cooked in boiling water until tender or done. This is the best method for cooking pasta, noodles, rice, and hard- or soft-boiled eggs.

- **Steaming.** Steaming is a healthy way to prepare vegetables. A small amount of water is boiled in the bottom of a saucepan and food is set over it on a rack. The pan is tightly covered to keep the steam in.

- **Poaching.** Fish or eggs may be cooked by poaching in barely boiling water or other liquid. Eggs are cracked and shells discarded before poaching. Fish may be poached in milk or broth, on top of the stove or in the oven in a baking dish.

- **Roasting.** Used for meats and poultry or some vegetables, roasting is a simple way to cook. Dry heat roasting means food is roasted in an open pan in the oven. Meats and poultry are basted, or coated with juices or other liquid, during roasting.

  Moist heat roasting is used for lean cuts of beef such as pot roast. Liquid such as broth, wine, or tomato sauce is poured over and around the meat and the pot is covered. Moist heat roasting may be done in the oven or on the stove top.

- **Baking.** Baking is used for many foods, including breads, poultry, fish, and vegetables. Baking is done at a moderate heat, 350°—400° F. Vegetables such as potatoes and winter squash bake very well.

- **Broiling.** Used primarily for meats, broiling involves cooking food close to the source of heat at a high temperature for a short time.

Meat must be tender to be broiled successfully. Inexpensive and lean cuts are often better cooked using moist heat.

- **Sauteing or stir frying.** These are quick cooking methods for vegetables and meats. Use a small amount of oil in a frying pan or wok over high heat.

- **Microwaving.** Microwave ovens are safe to use for defrosting, reheating, and cooking. However, "cold spots" can occur in microwaved foods. To minimize cold spots, stir and rotate the food once or twice during cooking. Place food in microwave-safe bowls before cooking. Never place metal thermometers or any metal object in microwaves.

- **Frying.** Frying uses a lot of fat and is the least healthy way to cook. Avoid frying foods for clients.

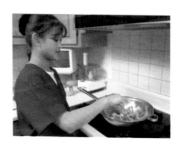

- **Fresh, uncooked foods.** Many fruits and vegetables have the most nutrients when eaten fresh, as in salads. However, fresh fruits and vegetables may be difficult for some clients to chew or digest.

GUIDELINES: SAFE FOOD STORAGE

- Buy cold food last; get it home fast. After shopping, put away refrigerated foods first.

- Keep it safe; refrigerate. Maintain refrigerator temperature between 36° and 40°F. Maintain freezer temperature at 0°F.

- Do not re-freeze items after they have been thawed.

- Use small containers that seal tightly. Foods cool more quickly when stored in smaller containers.

- Never leave foods out for more than two hours.

- Tightly cover all foods. Store with enough room around them for air circulation.

- To prevent dry foods, such as cornmeal and flour, from becoming infested with insects, store these items in tightly sealed containers.

- Check dry storage areas periodically for signs of insects and rodents.

- Check the expiration dates on foods, especially perishables.

- Check the refrigerator frequently for spoiled foods. Discard any you find.

Cooking Safety

- Do not cook with long, loose sleeves that can catch on pot handles or catch fire.

- Turn pot handles toward the back of the stove to prevent tipping.

- Dry hands before using electrical appliances.

- Immediately clean any spills on the floor to prevent slipping.

- When lighting a gas stove or oven, light the match before turning on the gas. Be sure the match is extinguished and cool before throwing it away. Never use a match to light a self-lighting gas stove.

- Store potholders, dish towels, and other flammable kitchen items away from the stove.

- Stay in or near the kitchen when anything is cooking or baking. Never leave stove on and unattended unless temperature is very, very low.

Assisting a client with eating

Equipment: meal, eating utensils, clothing protector if appropriate, 1-2 napkins or washcloths

1 Wash your hands.

2 Explain the procedure to the client. Speak clearly, slowly, and directly, maintaining face-to-face contact whenever possible.

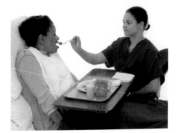

3 Assist the client to wash her hands if client cannot do it on her own.

4 Before assisting with feeding the client, see that client is in an upright sitting position (at a 90-degree angle).

5 Assist client to put on clothing protector, if desired.

6 Sit next to the client at the client's eye level. Sit on the stronger side if the client has one-sided weakness.

7 Check temperature of food. Offer the food in bite-sized pieces. Alternate types of food offered, allowing for client's preferences. (Do not feed all of one type before offering another type.) Make sure the client's mouth is empty before offering the next bite of food or sip of drink.

8 Offer drinks throughout the meal. If you are holding the cup, touch it to the client's lips before you tip it. Give small frequent sips. Use a straw or adaptive cup as necessary or as the client requests it.

9 Wipe food from the client's mouth and hands as necessary during the meal. Wipe again at the end of the meal.

10 Talk with the client during meal. It makes mealtime more enjoyable. Do not rush the client.

11 When the client is done eating, remove the clothing protector if used. Remove the tray or dishes.

12 Wash your hands.

13 Assist the client to a comfortable position.

14 Document the client's intake, if required, and any observations. How did the client tolerate being

upright for the meal? Did the client eat well? What foods did the client eat or not eat? Report any swallowing difficulties to your supervisor.

19. Managing Time and Money

Managing Time

Balancing your responsibilities means that you will need to learn ways to manage your time and energy efficiently. The following are ways to be sure your work schedule is as efficient as possible:

1 **Distribute tasks.** Look at the client care plan and your assignments. Note the assigned housekeeping tasks. Divide the tasks and schedule them for the week and the month. Make sure all your assignments can be completed in the time you have.

2 **Prioritize tasks.** Prioritizing your tasks is an important time and energy management skill. Think about the jobs and activities you want to get done throughout the day. Which ones must be done immediately? Which ones must be done at a certain time? Which activities are not absolutely essential and could be put off? Spend time on activities that are most important first.

3 **Simplify tasks.** Learn to simplify your tasks. Take time to think about how you will go about doing a task. Try to eliminate a few steps but still get the same result.

4 **Be realistic.** You may not be able to get everything done even if you plan carefully. When tasks take longer than you expected, or unexpected tasks need to be done, be realistic about what you can do. Do not be afraid to change your plan. Be flexible.

Many of the ideas for managing time on the job can be used to manage your personal time as well. The following are five basic strategies for managing time:

1 **Plan ahead.** Planning is the single best way to help you manage your time better.

2 **Prioritize.** Identify the most important things to get done. Do these first.

3 **Make a schedule.** Write out the hours of the day and fill in when you will do what.

4 **Combine activities.** Can you read the paper while you're on the bus? Work more efficiently when you can.

5 **Get help.** It is not reasonable for you to do everything.

Work Plan

The client care plan and your assignments will tell you what tasks are required. You can develop your own work plan. This will allow you to finish all your assigned tasks as quickly and efficiently as possible. For each day or block of time you will spend in a home, list all the tasks you must complete. Then, prioritize them. Mark the most important as "1" and the next most important as "2," and so on. Finally, write out a schedule for the day, filling in the highest priority tasks first.

Remember to distribute tasks evenly, so that you are not trying to do all the housecleaning on one afternoon and end up with no time to bathe or care for a client. Simplify tasks whenever possible to allow you to accomplish more.

Following an established work plan will also allow your clients and families to know what to expect of you. You may even want to discuss the plan with a client or family member as you are making it up or when it is finished. Some people appreciate knowing what will be happening in their homes at any given time.

Occasionally, you may be asked to do something that is not in the care plan or your assignments. There are several ways to handle requests that you must refuse.

1 Explain that you are only allowed to do tasks assigned in the care plan.

2 Explain that nurses familiar with the client's condition give you your assignments.

3 Emphasize that you would like to help, but you are limited to the tasks outlined in the care plan and your assignments.

4 Contact your supervisor after explaining these points. Your supervisor may add the requested task to your assignments. Be sure to document the client's request and the actions you took to address it.

Client's Money

Different states and employers have different regulations and policies regarding healthcare employees handling clients' money. Find out from your employer whether you will be expected to handle clients' money. If you are not allowed to handle money, never agree to do so, even occasionally. You could get yourself and your employer in serious trouble.

GUIDELINES: HANDLING CLIENTS' MONEY

- Never use a client's money for your own needs, even if you plan to pay it back. This is considered stealing.

- Estimate the amount of money you will need before requesting it. You may need to take things off your list or estimate the total bill as you go along in the store to stay within the money allotted.

- Take checks rather than cash, when possible. Have the client or family member fill out the name of the store. A signed check that is not made out is as good as cash.

- Get a receipt for every purchase. This proves how much you spent and gives a record for you and the client.

- Return receipts and change to client or family member immediately. Do not wait until the end of the day or week to settle up. Do it right away while everything is fresh in your mind.

- Keep a record of money you have spent. Follow your agency's policies for documenting money transactions. Write down how much you spent and where. Note any change returned to client. The better record you have, the smaller the chance of misunderstanding.

- Keep a client's cash separate from yours. If you must use the client's cash, do not put it in your own wallet. Keep it in a separate, safe place. Do the same with change. This will prevent confusion.

- Never offer money advice to a client. You should not even refer a client to others regarding their financial matters.

- Your clients' financial matters are confidential. Never discuss your clients' money matters with anyone.

VII
Caring For Yourself

20. Continuing Education

Each state has slightly different requirements for maintaining certification. Be familiar with the requirements. Follow them exactly or you will not be able to keep working as an aide. Ask your instructor or employer for the requirements in your state. Know how many hours of in-service education are required per year. You also need to know how long an absence from working is allowed without retraining or recertification.

Some states do not have a registry for home health aides like the ones they maintain for certified nursing assistants (CNAs). If, for example, you have taken the certification exam for CNAs and are on the state registry, you may need to work a certain number of hours in a long-term care facility to remain on the registry. As a home health aide, ask your employer how best to maintain your certification.

The federal government requires that home health aides have 12 hours of continuing education each year. Some states may require more. In-service continuing education courses help you keep your knowledge and skills fresh. Classes may also provide you with more information about certain medical conditions, challenges that you face in working with clients, or regulation changes.

Your employer may be responsible for offering continuing education courses. However, you are responsible for attending and completing them. Specifically, you must do the following:

- Sign up for the course or find out where it is offered.

- Attend all class sessions.

- Pay attention and complete all the class requirements.

- Make the most of your time during in-service programs. Participate!

- Keep original copies of all certificates and records of your successful attendance so you can prove you took the class.

21. Stress Management

Stress is the state of being frightened, excited, confused, in danger, or irritated. We usually think only bad things cause stress. However, positive situations can cause stress, too. For example, getting married or having a new baby are usually positive situations. But both can cause enormous stress because of the changes they bring to our lives.

You may be thrilled when you get a new job as a home health aide. But starting work may also cause you stress. You may be afraid of making mistakes, excited about earning money or helping people, or confused about how to perform your new duties. Learning how to recognize stress and what causes it is helpful. Then you can master a few simple techniques for relaxing and learn to manage stress.

A stressor is something that causes stress. Anything can be a stressor if it causes you stress. Some examples include:

- divorce
- marriage
- a new baby
- children growing up
- children leaving home
- losing a job
- starting a new job
- problems at work
- new responsibilities at work
- supervisors
- co-workers
- clients
- illness
- finances

Stress is not only an emotional response. It is also a physical response. When we experience stress, changes occur in our bodies. The endocrine system produces more of the hormone adrenaline. This can increase nervous system response, heart rate, respiratory rate, and blood pressure. This is why, in stressful situations, your heart beats fast, you breathe hard, and you feel warm or perspire.

Each of us has a different tolerance level for stress. In other words, what one person would find overwhelming might not bother another person. Your tolerance of stress depends on your personality, life experiences, and physical health.

GUIDELINES: MANAGING STRESS

- To manage stress in your life, develop healthy diet, exercise, and lifestyle habits.
- Exercise regularly.
- Eat a nutritious diet.
- Get enough sleep.
- Drink only in moderation.
- Do not smoke.
- Find time at least a few times a week to do something relaxing.

Stress can seem overwhelming when you try to handle it by yourself. Often just talking about stress can help you manage it better. Sometimes another person can offer helpful suggestions for managing stress. Sometimes you will think of new ways to handle stress just by talking it through with another person.

Try the following people and places for help with managing stress:

- your supervisor or another member of the care team for work-related stress
- your family
- your friends
- your place of worship
- your physician
- a local mental health agency
- any phone hotline that deals with related problems (check your local yellow pages)

It is not appropriate to turn to your clients or their family members to help you manage stress. One of the best ways to manage is to develop a plan for managing stress. The plan can include things you will do every day and things to do in stressful situations. When you think about a plan, you first need to answer the following questions:

- What are the sources of stress in my life?

- When do I most often experience stress?
- What effects of stress do I see in my life?
- What can I change to decrease the stress I feel?
- What do I have to learn to cope with because I cannot change it?

When you have answered these questions, you will have a clearer picture of the challenges you face. Then you can try to come up with strategies for managing stress.

22. Your Career

Specialty training for HHAs is additional training to prepare an aide to care for clients with specific medical conditions. When a person becomes specialized, he or she learns as much as possible about that type of care in order to offer more advanced skills than those taught in basic training programs. The specialty-trained HHA has more education and more experience than other aides. He or she will be a better prepared caregiver. If you are interested in specialty training, consider the following:

- Choose a specialty that you seem to be more interested in than any other. Doing what you like to do every day is very important.
- Choose a specialty that your agency has the most referrals for or that you know you can put to use in your particular area.
- Choose a program that is well-written and designed especially for your level of education and skills.
- Read as much as you can about this condition on your own.
- Discuss being assigned these types of clients with your supervisor.
- Talk to your clients who have this medical condition to gain some insight into their lives. Find out how they are affected from day to day.

After you are hired at an agency, there may be times you will need to make a complaint or voice a concern about some part of your job. Do not be afraid to do this, but do it carefully.

Think about the problem. Some major problems must be reported right away. For example, if a client, family member, or coworker threatens you, report this to your supervisor immediately. Other problems may work themselves out in time. If a new client seems rude, it is possible that he or she feels uncomfortable with new people or does not understand your role. You may want to wait several days or weeks to see if things improve before making a complaint. Know which problems should be reported immediately to your supervisor.

Plan what you will say. Think through and even write out what you will say to your supervisor. This will help you present your complaint clearly and completely.

Do not get emotional. Some situations may be very upsetting. However, you will be more effective in communicating and problem-solving if you can keep your emotions out of it. Share your feelings about a situation—whether you are mad, hurt, or annoyed—with a friend. Tell your supervisor the facts.

Do not hesitate to communicate situations that you feel are important or that may put you or a client at risk. One common problem in home care is aides not reporting when they feel unsafe at a particular client's home. In this case, not complaining can prove dangerous for you and the client. Always report to your supervisor any situation in which you feel you or the client is at risk of harm, even if the situation involves the client's family or friends.

If you decide to change jobs, be responsible. Always give your employer at least two weeks' written notice that you will be leaving. Otherwise, assignments may be left uncovered, or other aides may have to work more until the agency fills your spot. In addition, future employers may talk with past supervisors. People who change jobs too often or who do not give notice before leaving are less likely to be hired.

Look back over all you have learned in this program. Your work as a home health aide is very important. Every day may be different and challenging. In a hundred ways every week you will offer help that only a caring person like you can provide.

Do not forget to value the work you have chosen to do. It is important. For your clients, your work can mean the difference between living at home and living in an institution. It can mean living with independence and dignity versus living without. The difference you make is sometimes life versus death. Look in the face of each of your clients and know that you are doing important work. Look in a mirror when you get home and be proud of how you make your living.

An important life skill is being able to reflect on how you spend your time. Learn ways to fully appreciate that what you do has great meaning.

Few jobs have the challenges and rewards of home health care. Congratulate yourself for choosing a path that includes helping others along the way.

VIII
Appendix

Common Abbreviations

ā	before	**FBS**	fasting blood sugar	**po, p.o.**	by mouth
abd	abdomen			**pm, PM**	afternoon
ac, AC	before meals	**ft**	foot	**prn, p.r.n.**	as necessary
ADLs	activities of daily living	**FWB**	full weight-bearing	**Pt.**	patient
		GI	gastrointestinal	**q̄**	every
ad lib	as desired	**H₂O**	water	**q.i.d., qid**	four times a day
am, AM	morning	**h, hr**	hour	**R**	respirations, right
amb	ambulate	**hs**	hours sleep		
AP	apical pulse	**I&O**	intake and output	**ROM**	range of motion
b.i.d., bid	twice daily			**s̄**	without
BM, B.M.	bowel movement	**MI**	myocardial infarction	**SOB**	shortness of breath
BP	blood pressure				
BR	bedrest	**N/A**	not applicable	**S/S, S&S**	signs and symptoms
c̄	with	**NKA**	no known allergies	**stat**	immediately
C	Celsius degree			**TB**	tuberculosis
CA	cancer	**NPO**	nothing by mouth	**temp**	temperature
cath	catheter			**t.i.d., tid**	three times a day
c/o	complains of	**NWB**	non-weight-bearing	**TPR**	temperature, pulse, and respirations
CHF	congestive heart failure	**O₂**	oxygen		
CPR	cardiopulmonary resuscitation	**OOB**	out of bed	**URI**	upper respiratory infection
		OD	right eye		
CVA	cerebrovascular accident	**OS**	left eye	**UTI**	urinary tract infection
		p	pulse		
dx	diagnosis	**p̄**	after	**vs, VS**	vital signs
F	Fahrenheit degree	**p.c., pc**	after meals	**w/c**	wheelchair

Glossary

Acute—Intense and short-lived.

Adrenaline—A hormone that can increase nervous system response, heart rate, respiratory rate, and blood pressure.

Agitation—A state of being excited, restless, or troubled.

Alignment—A state in which the two sides of the body are mirror images of each other, with body parts lined up naturally.

Alzheimer's disease—A progressive and degenerative disease that causes dementia; there is no cure.

Angina pectoris—Chest pain.

Anorexia—A disease in which a person avoids eating or exercises excessively to lose weight.

Aphasia—The inability to speak or to speak clearly.

Apical pulse—The pulse on the left side of the chest, just below the nipple.

Arthritis—A general term that refers to inflammation of the joints.

Arteries—Type of blood vessels that carry oxygen-rich blood away from the heart.

Asepsis—A state in which no pathogens are present.

Aspiration—The inhalation of food or drink into the lungs; can cause pneumonia or death.

Asthma—A chronic inflammatory disease that makes it difficult to breathe and causes coughing and wheezing.

Body mechanics—The way the parts of the body work together whenever a person moves.

Bronchitis—An irritation and inflammation of the lining of the bronchi.

Catheter—A tube used to drain urine from the bladder.

Chronic—Long-term or long-lasting.

Colostomy—Removal of part of the intestine; causes stool to be semi-solid.

Combustible—Easily able to explode or catch fire.

Compassionate—Being caring, concerned, considerate, empathetic, and understanding.

Confidentiality—Keeping private things private.

Congestive heart failure (CHF)—A condition in which the heart muscle is damaged and cannot pump effectively; blood backs up into the heart instead of circulating.

Conscientious—Always trying to do one's best.

Constipation—The inability to have a bowel movement.

Constrict—To narrow.

Contracture—The permanent and often painful stiffening of a joint and muscle.

CPR (cardiopulmonary resuscitation)—Medical procedures used when a person's heart or lungs have stopped working.

CVA (cerebrovascular accident)—A condition caused when blood supply to the brain is cut off suddenly by a clot or a ruptured blood vessel; also called stroke.

Cyanotic—Skin that is pale or blue.

Dehydration—A serious condition that results from inadequate fluid in the body.

Dementia—A serious loss of mental abilities such as thinking, remembering, reasoning, and communicating.

Depression—An illness that causes withdrawal, lack of energy, and a loss of interest in activities, as well as other symptoms.

Diabetes—A condition in which the pancreas does not produce enough insulin; causes problems with circulation and can damage vital organs.

Diarrhea—The frequent elimination of liquid or semi-liquid feces.

Diastolic—Second measurement of blood pressure; when the heart relaxes.

Dilate—To widen.

Disorientation—Confusion about person, place, or time.

Draw sheet—An extra sheet placed on top of a bottom sheet; it allows repositioning of a person without causing shearing on the skin.

Epilepsy—An illness of the brain that causes seizures.

Ethics—The knowledge of right and wrong.

Evacuation—Leaving in an emergency.

Fracture—A broken bone.

Gastroesophageal reflux disease (GERD)—A chronic condition in which the liquid contents of the stomach back up into the esophagus; causes bleeding or ulcers and difficulty swallowing.

Glaucoma—A condition in which the pressure in the eye increases, damaging the optic nerve and causing blindness.

Hand hygiene—Handwashing with either plain or antiseptic soap and water and using alcohol-based hand rubs.

Hemiparesis—Weakness on one side of the body.

Hemiplegia—Paralysis on one side of the body.

Hepatitis—Inflammation of the liver caused by infection; can cause damaged liver function and other chronic, life-long illnesses.

HMO (health maintenance organization)—If you belong to an HMO, you must use a particular doctor or group of doctors except in case of emergency.

Homeostasis—The condition in which all of the body's systems are working their best.

Hormones—Chemical substances created by the body that control numerous body functions.

Hygiene—The term used to describe practices to keep bodies clean and healthy.

Hyperglycemia—A life-threatening complication of diabetes that can result from undiagnosed diabetes, not enough insulin, eating too much, not getting enough exercise, or stress; also called diabetic coma or acidosis.

Hypertension—High blood pressure.

Hypoglycemia—A life-threatening complication of diabetes that can result from either too much insulin or too little food; also called insulin shock.

Incident report—A report that must be completed when an accident or other significant event occurs during a visit.

Incontinence—The inability to control the bladder or bowels.

Infectious—Contagious.

Intravenous (IV)—Into a vein.

Laws—Rules set by the government to protect people and help them live peacefully together.

Lymph nodes—Oval-shaped bodies found in the neck, groin, and armpits that filter out germs and waste products carried from the tissues by the lymph fluid.

Medicaid—A medical assistance program for low-income people.

Medicare—Health insurance program for people 65 or older and people of any age who are disabled or ill and cannot work.

Metabolism—A body's physical and chemical processes.

Microorganism—A tiny living thing always present in the environment; not visible to the eye without a microscope.

Mucous membranes—The linings of the mouth, nose, eyes, rectum, or genitals.

Multiple sclerosis—A progressive disease of the nervous system in which the protective covering for the nerves, spinal cord, and white matter of the brain breaks down over time; without this covering, nerves cannot send messages to and from the brain in a normal way.

Myocardial infarction—A condition in which blood flow to the heart is completely blocked and muscle cells die; also called a heart attack.

Neglect—Harming a person physically, mentally, or emotionally by failing to give needed care.

Neuropathy—A nervous system disorder causing numbness, tingling, and pain in the feet and legs.

Nonverbal communication—Communicating without using words.

OSHA (Occupational Safety and Health Administration)—A federal government agency that makes rules to protect workers from hazards on the job.

Osteoporosis—A condition in which the bones become brittle and weak; may occur due to age, lack of hormones, lack of calcium, alcohol consumption, or lack of exercise.

Ostomy—The surgical removal of a portion of the intestines or urinary tract.

Pathogen—Disease-causing microorganism.

Perineal/perineum—The anus and genitals and the area between them.

Phobia—An intense form of anxiety or fear.

Physical abuse—Any treatment, intentional or unintentional, that causes harm to a person's body; includes slapping, bruising, cutting, burning, physically restraining, pushing, shoving, or rough handling.

Policy—A course of action to be followed.

PPO (preferred provider organizations)—A network of providers that contract to provide health services to a group of people.

Pressure sore—A serious wound resulting from skin breakdown; also known as decubitus ulcer or bed sore.

Procedure—A particular method, or way, of doing something.

Prosthesis—An artificial body part.

Psychological abuse—Emotionally harming a person by threatening, scaring, humiliating, intimidating, isolating, insulting, or treating him or her as a child; also includes verbal abuse.

Psychosocial needs—Needs involving social interaction, emotions, intellect, and spirituality.

Range of motion (ROM)—Exercises that put a joint through its full arc of motion.

Respiration—The process of breathing air into the lungs and exhaling air out of the lungs.

Schizophrenia—A brain disorder that affects a person's ability to think and communicate clearly, as well as manage emotions, make decisions, and understand reality.

Scope of practice—Defines the things a home health aide is allowed to do and how to do them correctly.

Sexual abuse—Forcing a person to perform or participate in sexual acts.

Specimen—A sample.

Sputum—Mucus coughed up from the lungs.

Stoma—An artificial opening in the body.

Systolic—First measurement of blood pressure; phase when the heart is at work, contracting and pushing blood out of the left ventricle.

Trochanter roll—A rolled blanket or towel that is tucked alongside the hip and thigh to prevent the leg from turning outward.

Tumor—A group of abnormally growing cells.

Validating—Giving value to or approving.

Verbal abuse—Oral or written words, pictures, or gestures that threaten, embarrass, or insult a person.

Table of Procedures

Our text includes numerous care guidelines. Please refer to specific topics in the index to locate them.

Index

Names and Numbers You Should Know

Abuse Hotline . . . .

Alzheimer's Association (local) . . . .

Area Agency on Aging . . . .

Church/Spiritual Advisor . . . .

Dietitian . . . .

Errand Service . . . .

Family Members . . . .

. . . .

. . . .

Fire Department . . . .

HHA Agency . . . .

Hospice . . . .

Meals on Wheels . . . .

Medical Supply Company . . . .

Natural Disaster Information Line . . . .

Pharmacist . . . .

Physician . . . .

. . . .

. . . .

Poison Control Center . . . .

Police Department (Non-Emergency) . . . .

Public Transportation . . . .

Senior Citizens' Center . . . .

Supervisor . . . .

Transportation Services . . . .

Other Resources: . . . .

. . . .

. . . .

. . . .

PRAISE FOR *CUTTHROAT*

"The family Sheffield: hugely rich and powerful—and murderously dysfunctional ... [T]he Brewer plotting is operatic ..."
—*Kirkus*

"Steve Brewer delivers a taut geopolitical thriller with sure-handed plotting and muscular prose. *Cutthroat* grabs you from behind, like a man with a knife who won't let go until he's done with you."
—Bill Fitzhugh, author of *Highway 61 Resurfaced*

"Steve Brewer hits the bullseye with a pulse-pounding page turner. *Cutthroat* is a lightning-fast read, a thriller that really thrills. Enjoy."
—Parnell Hall, author of *Hitman*

"Steve Brewer's *Cutthroat* is a classic suspense novel. Solomon Gage, taken in by the patriarch of the wealthy Sheffield family, is ferociously loyal and proficient in his role of troubleshooter. But the Sheffield family is up to its neck in trouble, and Gage can no longer protect the sons of the family from the consequences of their actions. All he can do is try to be the last man standing . . . *Cutthroat* is a terrific read and Brewer is a terrific writer."
—Charlaine Harris, New York Times bestselling author of *All Together Dead*

"Solomon Gage is the man I want watching my back. Brewer delivers on every level."
—*Crimespree Magazine*

ALSO BY STEVE BREWER

THE BUBBA MABRY MYSTERIES:
Lonely Street

Baby Face

Witchy Woman

Shaky Ground

Dirty Pool

Crazy Love

Monkey Man

THE DREW GAVIN MYSTERIES:
End Run

Cheap Shot

STANDALONES:
Fool's Paradise

Bullets

Boost

Bank Job

Whipsaw

NONFICTION:
Trophy Husband: A Survival Guide to Working at Home